T0033014

WIKIPENIS

WIKIPENIS

DR. NICOLA'S PENIS BOOK—
MAINTENANCE, PREVENTION, AND CARE

NICOLA MONDAINI
AND PATRIZIA PREZIOSO

TRANSLATION BY BRETT AUBERBACH-LYNN

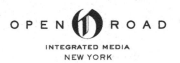

OPEN ROAD
INTEGRATED MEDIA
NEW YORK

All rights reserved, including without limitation the right to reproduce this book or any portion thereof in any form or by any means, whether electronic or mechanical, now known or hereinafter invented, without the express written permission of the publisher.

Originally published under the title *Wikipene. Manutenzione, prevenzione e cura*

Copyright © 2021 by Giunti Editore S.p.A., Firenze-Milano
www.giunti.it

Illustrations by Giulia Laino
Photograph on page 108 used with permission from Simone Mastrelli

ISBN: 978-1-5040-9401-6

This edition published in 2024 by Open Road Integrated Media, Inc.
180 Maiden Lane
New York, NY 10038
www.openroadmedia.com

To the patients, who have taught us that listening is the first medicine

CONTENTS

CONTENTS

PREFACE

Most powerful is he who has himself in his own power.

SENECA

I'm a woman and every Friday for the last few weeks I've been going to a urologist. An uncommon experience, to say the least. I walk in, sit down off to one side, and wait for Dr. Mondaini to finish his day's appointments. I usually pass the time correcting my notes, contemplating the posters on the waiting room walls in search of inspiration, or lazily browsing through the news on my phone.

When my gaze inadvertently moves around the room, I catch someone peering at me suspiciously. It might not be the first time they've seen me, they might want to ask me what I'm doing here. But they usually don't. Maybe one out of every ten speaks up.

If the book you're holding were a sociology treatise, we could analyze the various reasons why, as we grow older, human beings, and particularly those of the male sex, become more inclined to repress their questions. As boys, curiosity and an irrepressible desire to understand how the world works characterize and guide them. But over the years, as time becomes a scarcer commodity or maybe out of mere laziness, men cease to explore, investigate and more generally give voice to their queries.

Perhaps the reason for the silence of the people seated in front of me is unrelated to all that and stems, rather, from embarrassment. That just happens to be the reason this volume exists in the first place.

Its fundamental goal, in fact, is to free readers from excessive prudishness and a lack of information concerning the penis. People are always talking about it; no other part of the male body gets as much attention—think about art, daily conversations, language—where it's a common form of profanity—but even our email spam folder.

Not the torso, not the biceps, not the glutes. No, it's the penis.

It's talked about and its feats are celebrated to an extent comparable only to the general public's ignorance of its being, its evolution and its functioning.

This knowledge gap provided the spark that inspired *Wikipenis*.

If I had to choose two adjectives to describe Dr. Mondaini, it would be a tough choice between enthusiastic, fun-to-be-around and surprising, but the truth is that to define him you only need to tell the story of his professional career, which is also an excellent example of how life can take you down unexpected paths. Our meetings began with a conversation aiming to collect a significant number of answers, then turned into a systematic gathering of data and clinical experiences, which the doctor certainly doesn't lack, given that he's one of the leading experts in the field. We also decided to make room for the stories of numerous patients he's treated in twenty years of work, in anonymous form, a way of making the science more familiar and using the unfiltered stories of people who have already found answers to their questions to comfort those currently in the dark.

Our common aim is to offer everyone, not just adult men but also—indeed, perhaps above all—young males and the female universe, a learning tool for the healthy and correct care of the male genital system, the prevention of potential pathologies, and their treatment. Ideally, we are speaking not just to those directly concerned, but also to mothers and grandmothers, girlfriends and wives, who often find themselves at a loss when faced with the complex universe of possessors of penises.

My own work focuses on the communication strategies of complex organizations, and the part I love most is studying the professional reality with which I'm interacting and the fields it operates in. To provide appropriate solutions, I find it useful to be able to anticipate people's questions, and this is the approach that we've implemented in writing this handbook.

As a communications expert and someone with a strong inclination to satisfy my curiosity through further investigation, I sensed a knowledge gap as well as the temptation to fill it. This book arose to give voice to questions that often go unasked, but also to offer a reliable and easy tool for those who want to understand their body.

The chapters dedicated to the phases of life are divided into three parts—upkeep, pathologies and emergencies—in order to facilitate consultation.

The first chapter functions as an introduction, beginning with anatomical illustrations of our protagonist, describing how it's physically structured and the mechanisms by which it functions, and keeping in mind its dual role as a part of the urinary system and a reproductive organ.

Then, in four dedicated chapters, the evolution of the male member is analyzed over the course of a lifetime, from childhood to old age. With the passing of time, in fact, every single part of the human organism changes and it's important to understand how it does so in order to avoid being a passive victim of the process.

The information provided is detailed and scientific, pairing effective communication with specialized preparation and extensive clinical experience.

Wikipenis aims to eliminate all doubts and embarrassment. You can read it from beginning to end for an initial overall picture, then consult specific sections as circumstances dictate. In an age in which we find answers to everything at the speed of a distracted click, we believe it's important to revive the good habit of using an analytical table of contents.

But the long and the short of it is that it doesn't matter how you use it, but that you read it, because we're sure that doing so will help improve the quality of your everyday life.

Patrizia

WIKIPENIS

INTRODUCTION TO THE PENIS

HOW IT'S STRUCTURED AND HOW IT WORKS

Over the course of my studies I considered specializing in a variety of quite diverse fields: psychiatry, orthopedics, gynecology. It was this last one that had eventually convinced me. Already I could almost imagine myself managing the delivery room, with aching new mothers and panic-stricken fathers. But when it came time to sign up for the exam, something held me back. It was one of those moments in life when I sensed the lack of a good reason, an answer to the question "Why, exactly?" It was like I was no longer in control of my life.

One morning I had to take care of some bureaucratic errands related to admissions and I happened to walk into Careggi Hospital's Villa Monatessa, the location of the urology ward. The mere idea of spending my days examining testicles and penises and sticking my finger in patients' rectums to do prostate check-ups had seemed like an utterly crazy choice. Yet it was then that a part of my future became clear to me.

Just a few weeks later I chose to do my specialization at the school of urology run by Dr. Michelangelo Rizzo. I'd always been fascinated by the ways life decides to disrupt our plans, and now I'd suddenly gone from seeing nothing but vaginas to envisioning forests of flaccid and erect penises.

Coming from a family of doctors, I always thought I was somehow predestined for this job; I had never been someone who swam against the current "just because," like a person born into a family of judges who, out of spite, decides to rob banks. My grandfather Fulvio, a greatly beloved family doctor, was my role model. When he set off into the countryside at night for an emergency, he would shoot his gun off into the air to announce his arrival. My father followed in his footsteps, though he innovated when it came to informing patients of his presence. He too soon became a point of reference for the community, and he taught me how crucial personal contact and the doctor-patient relationship were to the profession.

When my two children had to describe their father's job for school, I had to think of the simplest and most effective way to clarify the meaning of "urologist." The first time I was caught off guard; the second time, I was ready. I defined myself as a "man's gynecologist." It's a paradox, but it's also easy to understand. In fact most, if not all, women turn to a gynecologist during their lifetime. But the same isn't true for men, who, knowing that they've been spared the travail of giving birth, consider periodic check-ups of their genitals to be unnecessary. As though the only reason for doing so had to do with the biological capacity to procreate.

The male equivalent of gynecology would actually be andrology, but doctors no longer specialize in this field. Andrology can be a concern for urologists and endocrinologists: while the former can operate directly on the patient, the latter deal solely with the medical and diagnostic aspects. Recourse to surgery is often necessary, which is why a urologist's comprehensive vision turns out to be useful. My work consists of both the medical and surgical component. I've come to love the line, "Penises pay my bills," from the famous song by Elio e le Storie Tese, though I certainly don't intend to compare myself to porn star John Holmes, the song's protagonist, famous for the size of his penis.

Urology and andrology are also my mission: with roughly two thousand examinations a year, I represent a source of information in a field still full of taboos and prudishness. For a decade I've been called to schools to examine boys, for a total of more than twenty-five thousand consultations. Emerging from this field work is the fact that one out of three boys has an andrological pathology. An astonishing statistic, if you think about it. Naturally, these also include the many small problems that can be treated as soon as they're identified. It's important to think of "treating" as a way of "taking care," preventing our minds from immediately racing to thoughts of drugs or invasive operations.

Before getting into the thick of things, we need to understand how a penis is formed and carefully analyze the parts of which it's composed. Human anatomy is a fascinating subject, but also quite complex. I still remember the nights I spent studying tables and diagrams, the wide-open windows in summer that brought in voices from the street as I reviewed hundreds of names of bones, muscles, tendons and systems for my university exams. Even after all that effort and over twenty years in the profession, I still consult anatomy volumes to track down this or that detail.

Truth be told, the time I found it most difficult to talk about penile anatomy was when Margherita, my eldest son Michele's fifth-grade teacher, asked me to make a presentation in class. It's difficult to simplify something without running the risk of trivializing it or taking it for granted, but today I can say that it was one of the most thrilling and stimulating teaching experiences I've ever had the honor to participate in.

Things exist for us in a whole new way when we learn to give them precise names, and the deepest knowledge stems from the correct association of names with their essence.

The penis holds a veritable record in the linguistic field. Between Italian and its dialects, colloquialisms and foreign imports, it's linked to almost seven hundred and fifty different terms, many of which are extremely expressive and certainly do it justice. There are countless nuances, ranging from weapons to the animal world to cooking implements and the emotional sphere, from ordinary legumes to the anonymous "member" of some unknown assembly, from "thingy" to "dick." In short, we risk getting started without a semantic consensus. What's more, many men are curiously reluctant to talk about their penises in any way that doesn't involve joking or teasing. So it's wise to clarify what we mean when we talk about the penis, partly to grasp a key element of our topic from the very beginning.

The penis is a quite peculiar, indeed a truly unique organ in the male human body. It is assigned a dual function: it's the final section of the urinary system, as well as the reproductive organ, a part of the genitals. This duality leads to its wearing two different "outfits": at rest it remains in a state of flaccidity, while in view of sexual activity it enters the state of erection, becoming rigid in anticipation of penetration. Describing it in these terms, it almost seems like a thinking organ, as you might have heard it referred to. It has a cylindrical, composite and variable structure. These adjectives immediately bring to mind the world of material science, and though this might seem remote, I guarantee you it isn't.

The penis was dissected and described for the first time by several Italian anatomists, including Falloppio and Vesalius, in the 16th century. Ever since there have been accurate renderings of its inner and outer parts, which we will use in this handbook.

Anatomically it is divided into three parts: the **root**, the **shaft** (or **body**) and the **glans**. Let's take a closer look at these components to gain a better understanding of how they function.

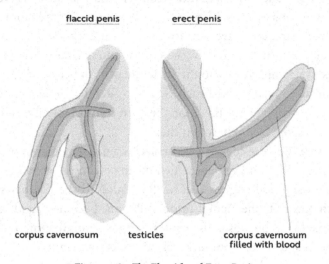

Figure n. 1—The Flaccid and Erect Penis

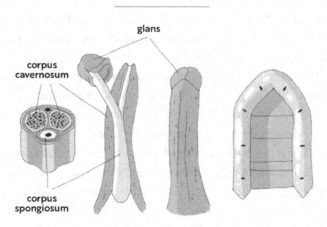

Figure n. 2—Anatomy of the Penis: Frontal section
and Resemblance to an Inflatable Raft

In order to visualize what we're talking about, it's useful to refer to images from daily life. I do an exercise with my students: I ask them to imagine the shaft's dissection in both directions, horizontal and vertical. And I can tell you that just thinking about it suffices to elicit more than a few pained expressions.

Inside the cross section are two lateral corpora cavernosa, separated in the center by the corpus spongiosum. The most effective comparison is to the structure of a rubber raft, like one of those you use at the beach. The two lateral cylinders are the hollow corpora while the floor, the most comfortable area, is the corpus spongiosum between them.

Traversing the **corpora cavernosa** is a network of minuscule cavities and blood vessels, which during erection become hard since the blood begins to flow. Returning to the comparison with the raft, the penis, upon inflation, becomes rigid and usable for its purpose. The central corpus **spongiosum**, on the other hand, is composed of elastic fibers and muscle tissue. Positioned in the direction of the abdomen, at its center lies the **urethra**, which connects the bladder to the external meatus. The human body is composed of extraordinary mechanisms and every tissue, vein, nerve or mucous is exactly where it needs to be, and nowhere else.

This apparatus of spongy and cavernous tissue protects the urethra, thus demonstrating the latter's importance. It's the urethra, in fact, that allows both for the release of urine when the urinary system is active and the release of sperm in the case of the genitals—the dual function of the penis we just mentioned. Unlike the more external cavernous cylinders, the corpus spongiosum, which doesn't fill up with blood, remains soft even during erection, allowing the urethra to maintain a certain mobility and facilitating the passage of liquids through it—semen or urine, as the occasion dictates.

These three elements are enveloped by a thin membrane, the **tunica albuginea**, with a unique composition. A series of collagen fibers arranged in strips render it an extraordinarily resistant structure, irrigated by blood vessels and reinforced by tendons, and covered in turn by other collagen strips alternating with elastic fibers: a sort of saran wrap for our meatloaf. It's this sophisticated and complex morphology, almost invisible from the outside, which explains the organ's variations in size and hardness and, above all, its resistance over time, despite the various stress factors to which it's subjected over the course of a life.

The penis thus composed is attached to the abdomen, and more precisely to the pubic bone, via the root. It's this non-visible part of the shaft that attaches to the three distinct points of the so-called urogenital triangle. Holding it all in place is the penis's **suspensory ligament**, a structure that is activated at the moment of erection so that the shaft tilts upward. It's what is known in engineering as a tie-beam.

At the opposite end of the organ is the summital part of the penis, called the **glans**, where the urethra's orifice (or meatus) is located. At rest, the glans is covered by a retractable strip of skin, the **foreskin**, connected to the shaft by a band called the **frenulum**.

At birth and for the child's first years of life, the foreskin remains closed to prevent the glans from coming into contact with feces and bacteria. After three years of age, it opens naturally. It can be removed via circumcision, but we'll talk about this in detail in the following chapters.

The male genital apparatus isn't composed of the penis alone, though this is undoubtedly its most "outgoing" organ. It includes other parts with varying degrees of visibility: the two **testicles**, two **epididymides**, two **vasa deferentia**, two **seminal vesicles**, the **prostate**, and the **bulbourethral glands**.

Put this way, its structure may seem similar to the plan of a house, in which each space performs its function but constantly communicates with the others. Indeed the penis could be the work of an extremely skilled architect, in which I, in the guise of a maintenance man, intervene to stucco cracked walls, fix broken locks, or change the wallpaper. So, just as you would for your home, you should turn to a urologist before the water heater breaks down completely and, most importantly, have your machinery checked periodically.

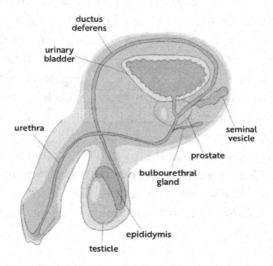

Figure n. 3—Complete Genital Apparatus

Part of this machinery are the **testicles**—also known as didymes—which resemble two olives and are contained in **scrotal sacs**, commonly called the scrotum. In an adult male they measure 3.5–4 centimeters in length, 2.5 centimeters in width, and weigh an average of 20 grams. These are the production facilities for spermatozoa and the male sexual hormones, known as androgens, which control the development of secondary sexual characteristics like the growth of the penis and the testicles themselves, the appearance of body hair, the enlargement of the prostate, and voice change. The production of these hormones begins with puberty.

There was a custom in the past, especially at Eastern and Chinese courts and in Ancient Rome, of removing certain young boys' testicles so their voices would remain high pitched. These castrated men—the eunuchs—were entrusted with supervising the harem because it was commonly thought that castration also led to the impossibility of having intercourse. In truth the lack of production of androgenous hormones and the lack of development of secondary sexual characteristics is reflected in various aspects of behavior and the body, but not in sexual ability: eunuchs could have sex, but it's likely they simply didn't feel the desire to, nor would they have been fertile due to their lack of spermatozoa and testosterone.

Above each of the two testicles is the spiral-shaped **epididymis**, which is simply a storehouse for spermatozoa. The epididymis connects each testicle to the **homolateral vas deferens**, a rather long canal of roughly 30 centimeters that represents the path the spermatozoa must travel to reach the urethra and thus leave the body.

But the voyage takes time. Before flowing into the exit duct, the spermatozoa must cross through the **prostate**.

The prostate is a gland positioned beneath the bladder and in front of the rectum. From the age of forty-five we should all regularly have our prostate checked via rectal examination. Not particularly looking forward to this event is more than understandable, but it's actually less traumatic than people fear and the benefits in terms of early diagnosis, reactive capacity and, last but not least, quality of life, are decidedly significant—we'll talk about this later on.

In normal conditions the prostate resembles a chestnut of roughly 20–25 grams, 4 centimeters wide and about half as thick.

Inside it, the spermatozoa are immersed in prostatic liquid thanks to the two **seminal vesicles**.

We might compare the seminal vesicles to the sight of a mountain lodge after a painstaking ascent: here, the spermatozoa receive nourishment (the prostatic liquid, like an armor protecting them from the elements, contains proteins, lipids, hormones, vitamin C and a great variety of enzymes without which the spermatozoa would die) and at the moment of ejaculation the vesicles push the liquid towards the exit point through the urethra. The sperm that comes out of the meatus at the moment of orgasm, in fact, is 90% prostatic liquid and just 10% spermatozoa.

Spermatozoa are those male reproductive cells that, during sexual intercourse, need to be in good enough shape to make their way up the female reproductive apparatus and fertilize the egg cell. To do so, however, there need to be at least fifteen million of them, only one of which will cross the finish line.

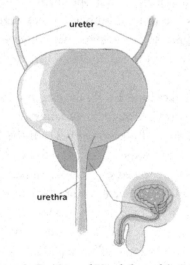

ureter

urethra

Figure n. 4—Position and Morphology of the Prostate

More than 90% of spermatozoa often present anomalies and thus are not fertile, but this needn't alarm us: even just a small percentage of spermatozoa with the correct morphological characteristics is sufficient for fertilization to occur. To evaluate our spermatozoa we can undergo a spermiogram, a test run after ejaculation that, with the help of a microscope, lets us verify the number, shape and mobility of the spermatozoa present in a specific quantity of seminal liquid. But be wary of do-it-yourself versions, which are often very imprecise; better to turn to a specialized laboratory.

The process of **spermatogenesis,** or the creation and maturation of the spermatozoa, occurs in the testicles' **seminiferous tubules** beginning with the onset of puberty and continues throughout our lifetime. Each spermatocyte contains 23 chromosomes, or half of the genetic information found in each human cell. The spermatocytes must mature and undergo various changes to become full-fledges spermatozoa; maturation takes roughly sixty-four days, but spermatozoa are produced continually. This replication process occurs though mitosis, or the splitting of the original cell, a process, however, which does not alter the number of chromosomes or the genetic information present, in a sort of multiplication pyramid. The mature spermatozoon fertilizes an ovule, which also contains 23 chromosomes: the result is in an embryo with 46 chromosomes. This union and the contribution of each parent determines the embryo's sex.

Before ejaculating, the penis produces a liquid known as **pre-ejaculate**. It lubricates the urethra to facilitate the semen's passage. Does it have the power to fertilize? The answer is no, for the simple reason that it doesn't contain spermatozoa, just prostatic liquid. So putting any doubts to rest, we can label it a natural lubricant that facilitates the functioning of our reproductive system.

At this point some of you might point out that I've yet to mention that question of questions, the one I've fielded the most since I got into this line of work. Briefly donning my architect's hat once more, I'm often asked about the **"standard size" of the penis**.

I have no precise and absolute answer because when we talk about the human body the adjective "correct" simply doesn't correspond to an equally univocal noun. Like all male physical characteristics, penises vary from person to person and we observe a great variety in their shape, color and size.

I've taken an in-depth look at the issue, particularly during my experience as medical officer at Florence's military recruiting center. At the time—it was 1998—scientific literature offered only one point of reference: the famous Kinsey Report from the late 1940s. Alfred Kinsey was an American biologist and sexologist who interviewed thousands of men and women to collect information about their sexual behavior. He also conducted a thorough study of the peculiarities and anatomical differences of the male gender. Yet his study was limited by the fact that it was based on asking men to measure their own penis with a common tape measure. The idea was interesting: this do-it-yourself approach could obtain a significant sampling of the population, and individuals were freed of the embarrassment of having to turn to a doctor. But the subjects involved, sometimes unconsciously driven by social pressure, ended up skewing the data upward for fear of being judged, and thus contributed themselves to fueling the myth of quantitative virility according to which the bigger the penis, the better. For years, then, the data were inaccurate and of no use for rigorous medical research: the study found that the male sexual organ was around 16 cm long on average, which is quite far from the reality.

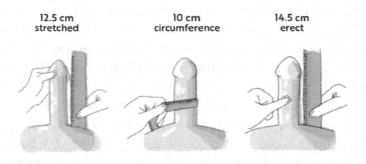

Figure n. 5—Average Penis Size by Circumference and Length

Penises are as similar in structure as they are infinite in their variety. Even Kurt Vonnegut, in his *Breakfast of Champions*, talks about the characters' penis size to give us an idea of how different they can be. He writes: "The largest human penis in the world was sixteen and seven-eighths inches long and two and one-quarter inches in diameter. The blue whale, a sea mammal, has a penis ninety-six inches long and fourteen inches in diameter." Pretty much the last word in the competition to see who's longest.

Over time, other attempts similar to Kinsey's tried to circumvent the obstacle of self-measurement by basing themselves on more objective foundations, but they ended up running aground due to the small size of the available data sample. The 1996 Wessels Study, for example, published in the prestigious *Journal of Urology*, the bible of American urology, certainly offered greater precision, but was limited due to the fact that its conclusions were based on a mere eighty patients.

Given this knowledge gap, I had the idea of taking penis measurements during the physicals I was conducting at the recruiting center—the opportunity was too good to pass up.

I disposed of a uniquely large research sample: twelve thousand young men born in 1980, in a single geographical area. I decided to focus on a random sample of three thousand three hundred subjects and took systematic measurements for an entire year. I thus created the **Penis Size Nomogram**, the standard of reference for penis length in European young men aged 18–20.

The results were quite different than those of the Kinsey Report. I measured the penis three different ways in an attempt to provide as complete an overall view as possible: when **flaccid** the penis measured an average of **9 centimeters**; when **stretched** (by pulling on the glans), it reached **12.5 centimeters**; when erect, roughly **14.5 centimeters**. As for circumference, meaning the distance around the shaft at its midway point, when flaccid it came to **an average of 10 centimeters**.

This "average" is important to remember. Being below or above the average, in fact, is neither a merit nor a demerit, nor is it something that conditions one's choice of partner.

One day I hope we will no longer consider penis size as an indicator of sexual satisfaction, as still happens far too often.

If you search the word "penis" on Google, the top results only seem interested in size, as opposed to health, hygiene and anatomy. "Women's preferred size," "national average penis size," "right size for man," "how to tell if he's well-hung," and "how to increase penis size with herbs" are only some of the suggested searches. One website (www.sizesurvey.com) claims to be the definitive collector of numerical data regarding penises, but it suffers from the same limitations as the Kinsey study; worst of all, its potential sampling is stuffed full of irritating ads about bizarre devices for penis lengthening, speaking volumes about its reliability.

Most men know the length of their own penis because in their teenage years—a time when insecurities are at their peak—they measured it with the help of a ruler.

But is such a measurement useful? The answer is definitely

no. Just as any correlation between penis size and foot length, hand size, height, nose, or any other part of the body is mere hearsay. They're false, remember that.

The obsession with size is rooted in time and history and widespread globally, regardless of nationality. Think about the penis-shaped amulets in art history books—there's even a branch of the subject dedicated entirely to the study of phallic symbolism, closely linked to the concept of fertility. But this is where you need to be careful: the concept of fertility must be distinguished from your partner's sexual satisfaction, potency, or muscular strength.

The size of the tool has nothing to do with a person's skill in lovemaking. A man who is sensitive to his partner's responses is a far better lover that one with a larger-than-average penis who makes love mechanically, as though it were a competition to see who can run farthest. And let me say one more thing: a large erection or large penis has no scientific correlation with greater fertility.

Maybe the ancients drew large penises simply to make them more visible from a distance . . . let's be thankful they decided not to use fluorescent paint, otherwise today's Google search results would include: "How to make your penis glow in the dark."

If you truly want a complete and truthful panorama of average penis size, visit a nudist beach rather than a porn site. Pornography often severely distorts reality: porn actors and the world that revolves around them are very distant from both what sexual intercourse is and the sizes of the body parts in question.

The lack of global data concerning penis size fuels many of the stereotypes presently in circulation: the Chinese are allegedly small, while there's no need to mention what people often assume about Africans. As I think is now clear from our analysis, generalization is a symptom of nearsightedness and insufficient preparation. In developing countries research is still behind, but progress is being made and perhaps in a few years we will have a comprehensive picture of the penises of all the world's ethnic groups.

Lastly, it's essential to underline just how unpredictable penises are.

The fact is that from the size of a penis at rest you can't extrapolate how much it will grow when erect. So be wary of competing against your teammates in the dressing room: don't assume you'll win easy, the results will surprise you.

Mothers' Needless Anxiety

I often have to reassure patients regarding the meaning of micropenis. Because of jokes, insults and unfair comments, this definition insinuates itself in the minds of those who think they're below the famous average we were just discussing. But sometimes it isn't the penis's owner who's concerned about its size, it's his mom.

"Good morning, doctor, this is Mattia and he's ten years old. I brought him to see you because his brother Tommaso, who's fifteen, had a much larger penis when he was his age. Could you give me your opinion?"

This is what passes for a greeting from the slightly heavyset woman with jet-black hair who's just walked into my office. Beside her, Mattia is looking at the photos on my desk. For him, none of what his mom said concerns him, or at least so it seems.

"There, see? Take a good look," the woman continues, after her son pulls his pants down.

After I take a quick look, she picks right up again: "So? Is everything okay?"

I carefully examine him and everything looks to be in order. Sure, his penis isn't large, but I refrain from saying this to the woman. In the presence of Mattia, who now seems bothered by my intrusion, words can suddenly become as crushing as boulders.

"Yes, ma'am, everything is as it should be. It's early to give a clinical judgment, Mattia is still young. Come back in two years and I'll be able to tell you more."

"Are you sure? I have to say, I'm a little anxious."

I had certainly noticed, but it's best not to mention this either. "Naturally."

I see Mattia again at thirteen. His mom has taken note of the changes and makes sure to give me her view: "Look, take a good look, it's gotten a little bigger."

The boy's penis is perfectly in the norm, it's simply taken a little longer to develop. We're accustomed to seeing boys take varying lengths of time to develop in terms of voice and facial hair; there's no reason it should be any different for the penis.

Today Mattia is eighteen, and no longer wants his mom along for the annual checkup. Last time I saw him he thanked me for having normalized the stress to which his mother subjected him at a very delicate time in his life.

Before leaving, he confides one last thing. "My girlfriend Ambra told me my penis is absolutely normal, not too big, not too small, just the right size."

Words can have a big impact on the psyche, whether it's a child or a young adult. This Ambra knows what she's talking about.

Between twelve and fifteen years of age, concerns regarding penis size are entirely premature except in specific and very rare cases. Between sixteen and eighteen, on the other hand, it's possible to formulate an objective evaluation of size and establish whether an individual is within the statistical norm or has what may be described as a micropenis. In medical terms, this expression defines the condition in which the flaccid penis is less than 3 centimeters long, and less than 6 when erect. I would add that this is actually a rare condition. Moreover, these measurements are purely indicative and must be placed in relation to height and body weight: a 10-cm penis can't be evaluated in the same way for a boy who's 1.49 m tall and a young man who's 1.92 m. Everything needs to be in harmony.

After speaking at length about the shape and size of our protagonist, let's dedicate a little space to the mechanism that makes it even more unique and amazing: **erection**.

At the foundation of the erection—the filling of the corpora cavernosa with blood—is a stimulus whose nature is entirely individual: it can stem from a visual, tactile, auditory, olfactory, even a psychological emotion. It's easy to think that it consists of a reaction to a naked body or the touch of a hand. But on closer inspection, an erection can be triggered by a few words, a particular smell or fragrance, or the briefest evocation of erotic thoughts. It's all subjective.

Reality is more complex than it appears. In a normal situation, one or more stimuli perceived at the conscious level activate the nervous system, which in turn transmits the impulse from the brain—or from the periphery, in the case of the penis's sensory receptors—to the erection's control centers, found in the lower half of the back at the height of the first and second lumbar vertebrae.

Here the impulses are reprocessed to provoke the release of neuromodulators, which allow the smooth muscle cells wrapped around the penis shaft to relax and, consequently, permit blood to flow into the corpora cavernosa. The latter function like sponges which, as they fill with liquid, increase in volume. Once triggered, the process is self-sustaining and the blood flow increases, giving the penis the rigidity typical of the moment of greatest arousal, which ceases only when the dilation of the corpora cavernosa ends up pressing on the vein and thus blocking the flow of blood. The corpus spongiosum also dilates during erection—as the name suggests, it's given to expanding following the absorption of liquid—though less so than the corpora cavernosa, so as not to occlude the urethra and to permit the passage of sperm during ejaculation. The corpus spongiosum is a sort of buffer state.

Ejaculation is the apex of arousal and of the sexual or masturbatory act, and is followed by a reduction in the amount of blood and in the pressure on the venous walls, causing the penis to be emptied and to return to its normal size—at least until the next time. After ejaculation, during which the heart rate reaches an average of 120 beats per minute, the penis experiences detumescence and goes into the so-called **refractory period**: a phase in which it isn't capable of achieving a new erection and can suffer irritation, even pain, if further stimulated, precisely because it has reached its maximum degree of sensitivity. This is a period whose duration varies and is tied to age: a healthy individual of twenty can experience a refractory period of just a few minutes, an elderly man of an entire day. For certain very rare subjects, this period lasts only a few seconds. Again, it's all subjective.

An important role in this process—particularly in relation to sexual desire—is played by the **endocrine system**, in charge of hormone production. A hormone is a messenger, like Hermes in Greek mythology: a chemical substance that's produced in a gland in a specific part of the body and then transported elsewhere by the blood. The **steroid hormones**—the **androgens**, one of which is **testosterone**—are produced in the testicles, regulate sexual desire and, in addition to influencing secondary sexual characteristics, participate actively in the erection. When the hydraulic and hormonal mechanism of the erection misfires—and let me repeat here just how crucial checkups are to avoid malfunctioning, the same as for a car engine—we have a case of **erectile dysfunction**, but we'll look at this in the coming pages.

Even in the absence of testosterone, or in situations characterized by its significant reduction, erections can still occur, particularly due to visual stimuli. For example, a transgender individual who is transitioning from man to woman, and is therefore undergoing a hormone therapy aimed at reducing testosterone levels as much as possible, can still have erections, with sexual desire remaining in the norm. Remember, testosterone is produced by the female endocrine system as well, though in far lower amounts than in a man.

Testosterone production is dictated by a circadian rhythm: it reaches its highest point early in the day, then falls as the hours pass. This is also one of the possible causes of the famous morning erections. Along with other hormones, it also has a role in spermatogenesis: for this reason hypogonadal patients—those with low levels of testosterone and testicles of a reduced size—often have problems linked to fertility. The production of male hormones diminishes with age, but it's a slow and gradual process, and never stops completely. There's no such thing as "andropause."

You've undoubtedly heard of the use of androgenous hormones in bodybuilding. Testosterone, in fact, is vitally important for the development of muscle mass, but it's important to avoid using it improperly and, most of all, to seek the guidance of a medical expert. One of the most common side effects of the unregulated assumption of testosterone is the obstruction of spermatogenesis, leading to a high rate of infertility and an increased likelihood of certain cardiovascular pathologies such as strokes. It's a risk that must be calibrated with great care.

Let's complete our picture with a discussion of the mechanisms linked to urination. How lucky we are that our tool is self-managing and spares us the worry of consciously performing these operations every time. Indeed, the more thoroughly we study the penis, the more complex and astounding it seems.

The impulse to pee begins in the **bladder**, which retains an increasing quantity of urine while keeping the muscle around the urethra's opening tightly closed. When the bladder nears full capacity, it sends signals to the spinal cord through the nerves of the pelvis, which generate a response impulse causing the contraction of the bladder and the muscle called the **sphincter** and allow the urine to flow out. Compared to erection, in this case we have greater control of the nervous stimuli from a very young age, learning to recognize them to free ourselves of diapers.

The penis's dual urinary and reproductive function is not just bizarre and curious but also extremely important, and characterizes the organ's dynamic, eclectic nature. Fundamental from the mechanical standpoint are the sphincters, the opening or closing of which activates one or the other system. Clinically speaking, we must always keep the penis's dualism in mind, particularly in case of a treatment or—even more so—operation that directly concerns it.

1

THE CHILD'S PENIS

"Dad, how do I wash it? Mom told me to ask you, since you take care of everybody's weenies."

"Well, not exactly *everybody's* . . ."

"So, can you help me?"

Childhood is the first age of man, a period of time that always seem too short to adults and too long to those going through it who can't do "grownup stuff." Of the many meanings that the term "growing" encompasses, one is certainly learning. Children are not miniature adults, but individuals with their own physical and intellectual peculiarities.

What we learn during childhood modifies the course of our existence and marks the contours of what we will be in the future. Our knowledge of and relationship with our body are thus fundamental elements for growing up healthy and happy.

This chapter aims to provide help and support to all adults who have the joy and responsibility of taking care of a little boy, accompanying his growth in an informed and conscious way, as well as to all those who simply have questions on the subject or wish to gain a more complete and coherent grasp of it.

After the announcement of a pregnancy, there are many questions that mom, dad, grandparents, aunts and uncles, second cousins and friends will ask themselves as they await the birth: Will the child be healthy? Will it get his nose? Her blue eyes? Uncle Stefano's bad temper?

But from the dawn of time, there is one that trumps all the rest: Will it be a boy or a girl?

I have met couples who, even before conception, looked into the suggested methods for having a boy or a girl, gathering suggestions and warnings from a wide variety of sources. You could write an encyclopedia on the sexual positions most appropriate for conceiving a girl, foods that are forbidden if you want a boy, and essential maneuvers for having twins, disregarding every study ever conducted on the laws of genetics.

While we're on the subject, I always remember the episode of the TV series *How I Met Your Mother* where Marshall and Lily are trying to decide on a name for their yet-to-be-conceived child, racking their brains over the pros and cons of having a boy or a girl. In the meantime, Marshall's father tells him that the reason the Eriksen family is made up of all males is due to their ancient Viking lineage. So, in keeping with his father's suggestions, before making love to Lily Marshall runs into the bathroom to eat pickled herring and dunk his testicles in freezing-cold water. And when he comes back to bed, he's careful to point his wife toward the north, the home of his ancestors. When Lily finds out about this, she reveals that she too had read up thoroughly on the subject. And when Marshall sees lemons on the side of the bed (which his father claimed were "fertilizer for females"), he realizes that she was trying to have a girl. In short, their plans would have canceled each other out and given chance the final say.

Couples wonder what their life will be like once the family gets bigger, and to gain a clearer view and soothe the concerns that parenting brings with it they make recourse to one of our most powerful weapons: the imagination. But this clashes with a lack of information about the newborn baby's sex, which amplifies and, simultaneously, diminishes the possibility of looking ahead to the various directions life can take. What's more, regardless of whether the future parents desire it or not, everyone will feel obliged to contribute to the construction of this image.

Grandma will immediately scrutinize the pregnant belly and pass judgment according to its shape: if it's more like a soccer ball it's a boy, if it's more elongated like a late-summer watermelon it's definitely going to be a girl.

Auntie will examine the future mom's body hair and, if it's increased, then "No doubt about it, it's a boy."

In no particular order there will be questions about the neo-mother's cravings—"Do you prefer sweet or savory?"—the temperature of her feet—"They're really cold, it's a he!"—and her morning sickness, with a precision of measurement worthy of the National Institute of Statistics.

I've heard them all: from a great-grandmother who convinced her granddaughter to tie her wedding ring to a string and position it over her belly and observe its oscillation (for the curious: if it swings back and forth it's supposedly a boy, while a circular trajectory indicates a girl) to ingesting a clove of garlic to verify whether the future mom is able to digest it. With tactics like these, it's no surprise that episodes of nausea are on the increase.

These popular beliefs get it right 50 percent of the time. They have no scientific basis, but it's clear that if you pick a random card out of a deck, sometimes you guess right. While some gurus go as far as to suggest the most propitious days of the week for having a girl, I feel confident in saying that the only secret there is to know is patience.

After clearing the field of voodoo rites and sacrifices to the pagan gods, after consulting the proverbs of every world region and studying the relevant spells and charms, it comes time for the long-awaited ultrasound. A child's **phenotypic sex**, or the presence of a penis and scrotum in the male and the labia majora in the female, can be diagnosed with reasonable certainty from the twelfth week of pregnancy.

Up to the seventh week of gestation there are no identifiable developmental differences linked to sex, though there actually are various diagnostic techniques that can be used beforehand.

Some of these are more invasive, such as **Chorionic villus sampling** at the tenth week, the now-obsolete **cordocentesis**, and **amniocentesis**.

The **NIPT** (Non-Invasive Prenatal Test), on the other hand, is of the non-invasive variety and consists of drawing blood from the mother, through which it's possible to attribute the **genotypic sex**—determined by the combination of two sexual chromosomes X and Y (XY for a male, XX for a female)—and identify other significant chromosomal anomalies. Genotypic sex and phenotypic sex coincide except in rare cases, but ultrasonographic attribution remains fundamental, a crucial moment for the determination of the child's sex.

At the twelfth week the penis becomes visible and measures 3–4 mm. In this phase it's very difficult to establish the presence of morphological pathologies in the shaft, but expert hands can already distinguish certain of them, like hypospadias.

But it will only be the obstetrician, at the moment of birth, who establishes the newborn's sex and points out any clear defects or genital ambiguities.

Fat Doesn't Steal, It Conceals

After discovering the sex, overcoming the travails of pregnancy, and making sure that the baby has his weenie, it seems like smooth sailing. That isn't exactly the case.

While I'm on my way to Catanzaro, where I teach at the university, the screen in my car informs me of an incoming call from an unknown caller. It happens quite often and I have to say that only two-thirds of them are telemarketers: they're mostly moms and dads who I don't know yet, but who are worried enough to turn to me.

"Hello, doctor, is this a good time for you to talk? We haven't met, I got your number from friends. If I may get right to the point, my son Alessandro has lost his penis, I need to see you as soon as possible."

In her voice I sense the drama she's going through and something worries me. Paola comes across as someone who's not so much anxious as she is extremely concrete. Without beating around the bush, in fact, she tells me she suspects that her son has ambiguous genitals and that, above all, his penis hasn't developed correctly. I reply firmly that I will certainly see them as soon as I return.

On Wednesday of that same week, in Florence, I meet Paola and her husband Pietro, who have come, however, without their son, who's at pre-school. They tell me about Alessandro and from their words emerges a normal boy of three who plays with his classmates, is very affectionate to his parents, is learning to communicate his feelings, and loves having goodnight stories read to him. A more than normal situation, I'd say, which limits my comprehension of the situation even further. It seems unlikely that his penis has retracted to the point of disappearing almost completely.

I meet Alessandro a week later, and I notice a detail that Paola and Pietro had omitted: Alessandro is obese. Now things start making sense.

Without mentioning it I have him get undressed and lie down on his back, while the two adults await my verdict. I place the palm of my hand on his pubic region and push down, the belly disappears and, as though by magic, out comes the penis. They look at me, I look at them.

They smile and scoff at one another. "How's it possible? How could we not have realized it? It seemed to have disappeared."

Without mincing words I explain to them that the problem isn't the disappearing penis, but Alessandro's weight. They confirm that he eats in a very disorderly fashion: cookies, milk, penne with tomato sauce and then again from the top, at every meal. At pre-school he refuses vegetables and fruit of any kind. In fact they too admit to not following a very balanced diet and that this has repercussions on the health of their son, who has very high cholesterol.

Alessandro has what's known as a "buried penis." The excess fat in the pubic region conceals, partially or wholly, the penis.

At this point I become categorical. "The problem, even if might not seem so to you, is more serious than expected: an overweight child will be an overweight adult. Even if his penis is still there and this concern has been resolved, there's no time to waste: all three of you need to see a nutritionist!"

"What do you mean, all three of us!?" Pietro exclaims in amazement.

"That's right, all three of you," I repeat, "a healthy diet needs to become your lifestyle because Alessandro has you as his example. A good diet needs to become an integral part of your family." Several months later, Katia, the nutritionist I had suggested to them, tells me that Alessandro and Paola are on the right track, but Pietro, after a promising start, has slacked off. But Katia isn't giving up.

Sometimes the solution is simpler than we think.

A buried penis is a problem of excess fat, which ends up "suffocating" the organ. Those who suffer from it are typically obese children, who in Western countries now account for 30 percent of the total. So the first step to take is to modify the child's diet: the loss of excess fat will guide the penis back out, as well as save the child from obesity and its related diseases, first among them diabetes. As we shall see, diabetes is the cause of even more serious problems, such as erectile dysfunction, phimosis (a condition we will discuss) and a greater predisposition to infections of the genitals and urinary tract.

UPKEEP

In this volume we've decided to dedicate significant space to the good practices for maintaining a healthy penis, which is why you'll often find me donning the shoes of the cautioning doctor, the apprehensive parent, and the friend who knows what he's talking about. As far as hygiene is concerned, during the first year of life it's advisable to wash only the outside of the penis using delicate soaps: those used for giving the baby his bath are fine. At the same time, diapers should be changed frequently to prevent irritations and dermatitis caused by a moistness and rubbing. While changing diapers, you've probably been hit by a spurt from the little boy's fountain: this occurs due to the change in temperature, which increases the stimulus to urinate, so be quick to take cover. In children, the foreskin is usually extensive, to protect the penis inside it in this very delicate phase of growth.

Early on, you should avoid the operation of **foreskin retraction**, which in addition to being painful could cause tiny cuts that, with scarring, create adhesiveness and the formation of a **phimosis**. In this period the glans is never uncovered, precisely because there is no need to. On the tip of the penis you might notice a whitish residue, called **smegma**, composed of dead cells and secretions. Remove this substance with great care and delicacy, because its accumulation can become fertile terrain for bacteria.

The scrotal area must also be cared for and cleansed with the same attention. It's also important to be sure that the genitals are dry at every diaper change, to avoid irritating sores. Our grandmas used clouds of talcum powder, but today a clean wipe or some starch will suffice.

Improper hygiene can be the cause of **balanoposthitis**, an inflammation of the glans and foreskin, on which staphylococci and streptococci proliferate. The glans and foreskin appear reddened, sometimes with swelling. The child manifests the need to urinate often and feels pain or burning while doing so. This condition, after identifying the type of infection, is resolved by applying antibiotic or antimycotic creams.

A final recommendation concerns caring for the child's genitals at the beach. It's a good habit to have a dry change of bathing suit, rinse the child off with fresh water after he goes in, and take care that the boy's weenie not enter into direct contact with the sand.

At twelve months, at bath time you can begin to slide the foreskin back, delicately and without forcing it, and remembering to return it to its original position—this step is fundamental for preventing accidents. Only around three years of age does it become a good idea to check that the foreskin is beginning to open naturally on its own.

At the age of four or five the child begins washing his penis by himself. This is the time to teach him how to do so, sliding the foreskin back when he cleans his genitals and every time he pees, to prevent drops of urine from stagnating under the foreskin, causing inflammations or infections.

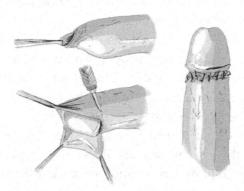

Figure n. 6—The Three Phases of Circumcision

Speaking of peeing: is it good to do so standing up as soon you're tall enough to use the toilet? The answer by and large is yes, since in males this is the only way for the bladder to empty itself completely. Residual urine, over time, could cause infections to develop.

It's also a good practice, at least early on, to go to the bathroom not just when the need becomes urgent, but with regularity, so as not to overload the bladder and cause it to lose elasticity.

I know that some moms will curse me for insisting on the need to pee standing up from a young age, but they ought to see it as an opportunity to teach their son to raise and lower the toilet seat, obviating the need to repeat it ad nauseam in the growing years (and beyond . . .). Plus, as everyone knows, we're more receptive at a young age.

Circumcised penises are a separate matter. First of all it's necessary to be clear about what we mean by **circumcision** and why it's practiced. This is a subject that touches on many fields and medicine is only one of them, not even, in my view, the most important. The decision to circumcise a newborn boy, in fact, is almost always made without the request for or the expression of a medical opinion.

Circumcision is a practice born in ancient times for essentially hygienic reasons. The peoples who practiced it lived in desert regions characterized by the outsize presence of sand and wind. In such a scenario, circumcision aimed to protect the penis from possible infections, since it reduced the risk of infectious agents being deposited between the foreskin and the glans. Over time the hygienic-sanitary imperative lost importance, partly due to improved living conditions, while the procedure's ritual meaning was maintained.

For Jews, circumcision takes place on the eighth day after birth and is a rite accompanied by ceremonies and blessings; it is said to represent part of the covenant with God, who in the Book of Genesis tells Abraham, "You shall circumcise the flesh of your foreskin."

It's a widespread practice among Muslims as well, but with a different, more discretionary calendar, often immediately after birth and in any case prior to puberty, while in the case of a convert it takes place just before his wedding. The religious belief at its foundation is that an uncircumcised man is not deemed worthy of entering heaven. In certain animistic religions as well the practice has a meaning of purification and passage, a common denominator in the various creeds.

Today, roughly 30 percent of the global male population is circumcised. In the United States the percentage surpasses 80 percent: quite peculiar, given that it isn't linked to religious reasons but to custom: "If people have always done it, then let's continue to do it." Some studies trace this practice back to the beginning of the last century, when circumcision represented a status symbol, a way to demonstrate that the family could afford to have the child born in a hospital. Yet again, its symbolic rather is prioritized over its medical value.

In clinical terms, circumcision is a surgical intervention that aims to remove the foreskin that covers the glans when it's over-abundant and unable to slide normally. From a surgical standpoint, it's justified in treating phimosis or contrasting other pathologies, such as balanoposthitis or serious, even chronic forms of urinary tract infection.

The operation, lasting roughly thirty minutes, is simple, but must only be carried out in a sterile, hospital setting. It calls for local anesthesia for adults and general anesthesia for young patients, to prevent the risk of sudden movements. The stitches fall off on their own without leaving a mark, with complete healing in roughly one month. Applying Vaseline for two or three days is recommended, to prevent the glans or the stitches from adhering to clothing in any way.

But we shouldn't lose sight of the fact that, except in specific cases, this is a non-necessary operation. Especially since in recent years there has been an increase in hospitalizations and even of deaths due to complications from these interventions, often conducted by unqualified personnel and in inappropriate locations, with consequent hemorrhages and infections. This is the reason why, due partly to the significant number of arrivals in Italy of immigrants from Muslim and Jewish countries, the National Federation of Doctors and Dentists has advanced the request to include ritual circumcision among the services provided by the National Health Service, to be carried out following the binding agreement of the doctor and payment of the copay fee. It's thus possible to regulate its practice and keep its effects under control. At present the project is still in the experimental phase and only certain hospitals—such as Turin's Maria Vittoria Hospital—have opened a multidisciplinary clinic for ritual circumcision. As an alternative, it is of course possible to turn to paid private institutes and clinics, which perform the intervention in conditions of maximum safety.

No international medical organization supports circumcision as a hygienic measure or good health practice, but it's true that none of them forbid it. Let's say that, outside of the therapeutic realm, it's a sort of custom, with some moderate benefits and few drawbacks when carried out correctly.

Tradition holds that circumcision reduces the risks of penile cancer, infant urinary infections and, later, sexually-transmitted diseases. The last two benefits can be obtained with simple and correct daily hygiene, but it's true that the risk of contracting STDs, above all HIV, is drastically lowered. This certainly doesn't mean that a circumcised male is immune from contagion and can afford to have unprotected intercourse, but that his likelihood of being infected is lower than that of an uncircumcised man. It has been demonstrated, however, that behavioral factors have far more impact in lowering the risk of sexually-transmitted diseases than any removal of that little piece of skin. In the past the World Health Organization has sent out recommendations explicitly in favor of the intervention, at least for certain regions of Africa. In this context, the WHO also supported a program for the introduction of devices making it possible to carry out circumcision in just over thirty seconds. The problem is that such tools have unsustainable costs even in Western countries, thus making them totally unfeasible for countries with emerging economies.

Regarding the subject of penile cancer, circumcision becomes necessary or recommended only in those countries in which a high number of people are still affected, such as in South America, where it accounts for 10 percent of all tumors in the male population. This occurs when male genital cancer is linked to a quite frequent infection, that of the Papilloma Virus. Roughly 70 percent of young men between twenty-five and thirty are believed to have come into contact with it at least once.

Insufficient hygiene thus becomes a real trigger. It's clear that, in these conditions, the likelihood of contracting pathologies linked to insufficient hygiene becomes extremely unlikely if the patient is circumcised as a baby.

Adult circumcision occurs only in cases of extreme necessity and can be more traumatic, particularly on a psychological level, than it is for a child.

PATHOLOGIES

The penile pathologies that are crucial to be on the lookout for from the first years of a child's life are cryptorchidism, hypospadias and frenulum breve.

Cryptorchidism

By **cryptorchidism**, also referred to as "testicular retention," we mean the failure of one or both testicles to descend into the scrotal sac. In these cases, the missing testicle has gotten "stuck" at some point on the journey it makes during the life of the fetus. The testicles, in fact, develop in the abdominal cavity, like a female's ovaries, before descending into the scrotum in time for birth. This isn't a total absence of testicles, but rather of an incomplete process of "descent." In roughly 50% of cases the condition resolves itself naturally within the first year of life.

It's important to verify, in a clinical setting and via MRI, whether the testicle is entirely absent or simply positioned at a point other than its natural one. In the latter case, it's best to operate to reposition it in the right location, or there could be serious risks both for the person's fertility, and of developing types of tumors. Hormonal therapy is the suggested approach. If administered within the first eighteen months of the child's life, it can resolve the problem. Should this not be sufficient, it's necessary to proceed to a surgical laparoscopy—technically referred to as an **orchidopexy**—which avoids incisions. If for any reason shifting the testicle to the proper location isn't possible, it's preferrable to remove it to avoid the risk of developing tumors.

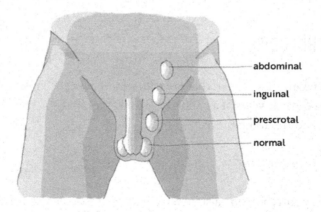

Figure n. 7—**Testicular Pathologies: Types of Cryptorchidism**

It's worth knowing that there's also a frequent condition known as a **retractile testicle**, in which the testicle, perfectly formed and situated in the scrotum, tends to move up, creating the visual impression that it has almost disappeared (it happens, for instance, with low temperatures). In this case cryptorchidism has nothing to do with it! The scrotum's volume changes continually over the course of our lives since the sac has a fundamental role in testicular heat regulation—it functions like one of those thermal blankets we see on television that resemble aluminum paper. Its task, in fact, is to increase or reduce heat dispersion as circumstances require. So always let a doctor examine your genitals and avoid self-diagnoses . . . let Alessandro and his buried penis be a lesson to us.

The opposite case is also possible, meaning that a child is born with more than two testicles, but this is an extremely rare condition, **polyorchidism**, resolved surgically with the removal of the excess testicles. The same can happen with the penis: it's possible, and I underline *possible* and not probable, to be born with two penises, in which case the correct term is **diphallia**. In most children affected by this malformation, urine and semen only come out through one of the two. This is an extremely rare condition, which statistically occurs in one in every six million males. Surgical removal of the excess penis is the only solution, and it's necessary, particularly given the psychological impact that a condition like this can have on the boy, first as a child and then as an adolescent.

Hypospadias

In the chapter on the anatomy of the penis we mentioned the urinary meatus, the small orifice present on the tip and out of which comes, depending on the system in use, urine or semen. It can occur, however, that the meatus is not located exactly at the end of the glans, but shifted toward the abdomen, known as **hypospadias**. This pathology is quite rare; according to one of my early studies, now twenty years old, it affected roughly 0.3% of the male population, though this doesn't mean it can be neglected. Urology textbooks report that the most famous man to suffer from it was King Henry II of France, husband of Catherine de' Medici. There is no proof of any repercussions on fertility.

The shift of the meatus is often associated with the appearance of a fibrous band that causes the penis to curve. Added to this in some cases is an anomalous distribution of the foreskin, with more skin on the upper (dorsal) part than below (ventral).

Cases of hypospadias are medically classified as first degree (the least serious), second degree and third degree, according to how far the meatus is from its ideal position at the tip of the glans. So there are extremely slight forms of hypospadias, in which the defect is difficult to even detect, and more serious forms that cause great discomfort.

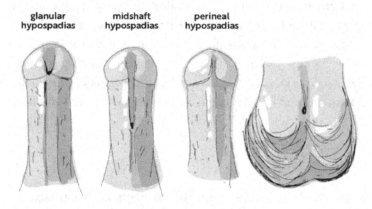

glanular   midshaft   perineal
hypospadias   hypospadias   hypospadias

Figure n. 8—Types of Hypospadias

If, for example, the meatus is not located at the tip of the penis but halfway down the shaft, the child cannot urinate standing up but must do so sitting down; if it is even lower down, at the level of the testicles, the situation becomes more serious. In this instance a more thorough genetic analysis is certainly appropriate: there are conditions in which children who appear male, but with an anomalous penis and without testicles, are actually genetically female. These, of course, are very rare events that conceal pathologies linked to phenotype.

The causes of hypospadias often have genetic origins, but can also arise due to environmental factors: it can be passed down from father to son, or caused by contact with toxic substances. Certain medications—and these include forms of birth control, perhaps taken by the mother during the first months of pregnancy—or specific chemical substances such as pesticides are possible determinants. Surgery is necessary to resolve the issue.

The operation should ideally be carried out prior to three years of age, before the child is aware of the situation and there's no risk of psychological trauma. If, on the contrary, you avoid dealing with the situation and years go by, complications can arise. In a clinical setting cases of hypospadias are treated by pediatric urologists with a precise specialization. The simpler ones require one, relatively simple operation, but more complex cases can call for several interventions, until the desired result is achieved.

To me, the key role of adults and parents in these delicate years appears even more evident in this light. Theirs is an essential function, in which observing and reporting is even more important than any assistance in treatment. So, especially in the early years of a boy's life, keep watch over the penis.

Frenulum Breve

Another congenital pathology is **frenulum breve**. The frenulum is the thin band of tissue that connects the glans to the foreskin and that performs an essentially mechanical function: the protection of the summital part of the penis. During erection, the foreskin slides back along the shaft until the frenulum intervenes to prevent it from pulling back to far. With the return to a state of rest, it pushes the foreskin back out and facilitates its return to its original position, functioning just like a rubber band. During sexual intercourse, on the other hand, it acts as a sensor: rich in nerve receptors, it transmits both the pleasant sensations of contact as well as any painful or unpleasant ones, as in the case of violent handling.

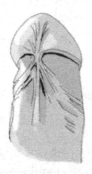 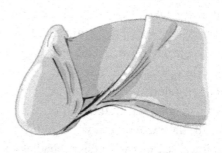

Figure n. 9—Frenulum breve

If this portion of skin is shorter than necessary, the foreskin may be unable to stretch out completely and be forced to fold downwards.

In this case there are three options. The first is to wait: do nothing, in the hope that the problem resolves itself naturally. The risk of waiting is that the frenulum could suffer lacerations, perhaps during sexual intercourse. This is a rather traumatic solution to the problem, because it provokes bleeding which, even if minimal, could cause panic. Alternatives include lengthening it surgically, or else performing circumcision. Most times—particularly in the case of small children—the latter option is chosen.

The operation to lengthen the frenulum, lasting roughly ten minutes, calls for the incision of the "thread" either with a traditional scalpel, followed by the application of several stitches that fall off by themselves, or with an electric scalpel, which cauterizes immediately and requires no stitches. Average healing time is around fourteen days, during which it isn't even necessary to protect the area with gauze or bandages. Daily medication is sufficient, consisting in pulling back the foreskin to expose the shaft and disinfecting the area with a liquid antiseptic or antibiotic cream. During recovery, the child may wake up during the night complaining of discomfort. This is natural and occurs because during sleep there are spontaneous, involuntary erections that pull on the incision area and thus cause pain.

Penile Curvature

Congenital penile curvature is a pathology of which it's important to evaluate both the physical and psychological significance. The condition concerns the axis of the penis shaft, which instead of being straight is tilted upward, downward or to one side, generally due to the asymmetry of the two corpora cavernosa. Of course a slight curvature is not to be considered problematic, but rather normal, as the human body is never symmetrical. It's necessary to operate, however, when such curvature exceeds 15–20 degrees.

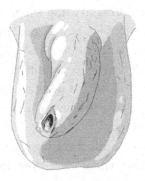

Figure n. 10—Penile Curvature

Congenital penile curvature is hardly rare—it's found in roughly 1 percent of boys—and can be diagnosed from early childhood. The difficulty lies in the fact that in order to diagnose it the penis must be erect. Which is why the first one to notice it is usually a parent, when the first spontaneous erections occur or during the child's bath. So set aside any useless prudery and pay close attention.

The only solution here is surgery. The operation can be done in the first years of the child's life—even prior to three years of age—but more often people decide to wait until after the age of sixteen, when the penis is already almost completely formed. It is difficult, however, to indicate a single, ideal period of time: many factors must be considered in each case, first among them, as we said, the psychological impact on the child.

The risks of an operation prior to three years of age are linked, in fact, to the penis's underdevelopment, and this is connected to the danger of causing a shortening which is then difficult to correct. Even if a congenitally curved penis—when not associated with other pathologies—is actually a longer-than-average penis, and thus an operation that might cause a slight shortening wouldn't have negative consequences in physical terms, it's important to closely consider and not underestimate the psychological implications.

Penile curvature, furthermore, has no effect on fertility. Unfortunately, however, it's a condition that is often kept hidden until adulthood, with a negative impact on sexuality. A crooked penis causes insecurity and fragility which, if concealed, are amplified.

Difficulties and discomfort during intimacy, lack of pleasure and even tensions with one's partner are all consequences linked to this condition. In reality, the solution to the problem is simple and fast: the straightening operation is now generally carried out in an outpatient context and full recovery doesn't take long.

Webbed Penis

A very rare condition concerning the penis's shape is webbed penis, manifesting itself as a strip of scrotal skin attached to the penis shaft.

Here, too, the solution to the problem is quite simple, since a simple surgery is sufficient to "detach"—and then remove— the excess scrotal tissue. The operation is brief, roughly thirty minutes, but requires caution in the recovery period. The penis, in fact, must remain covered and be disinfected daily for a certain period. It is thus best to plan this type of surgery far from the summer period, because contact with sand and seawater can lead to complications.

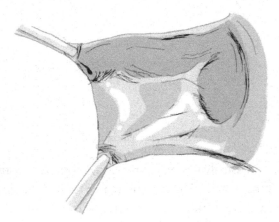

Figure n. 11—Webbed Penis

Phimosis

We've learned that even the scariest pathologies for the child and the parents can be resolved without excessive difficulty. The same is true for phimosis, when the foreskin covering the glans doesn't open naturally, as it should on its own around age three with the abandonment of diapers—which is why we can only speak of phimosis from the age of 3–4.

If phimosis is congenital—present, that is, from birth—I suggest, on the one hand, using creams that facilitate the normal sliding of the foreskin and, on the other, delicately pulling back on it, perhaps at bath time, to facilitate its opening. Practicing, that is, a sort of foreskin stretching, helping it realize its potential.

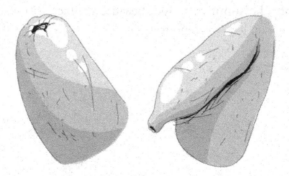

Figure n. 12—Phimosis

Phimosis is usually resolved this way, without further medical care. But if these manual interventions aren't sufficient, surgery is necessary. In this case the solution is circumcision, performed by a pediatric urologist, which completely eliminates the constriction.

An operation must also be considered in cases of **acquired phimosis**, or those pathological forms that aren't present at birth but arise over time, and which can be the consequence, for example, of genital infections or dermatitis. These forms are quite rare in children, but they mustn't be excluded and have to be quickly and correctly treated.

Varicocele

Unlike webbed penis, **varicocele** concerns the testicles and particularly their vascular system. It can appear from the initial stages of a child's life and becomes more significant during puberty and adulthood: indeed it's often asymptomatic, only identifiable through a routine checkup.

A precise diagnosis can usually only be made starting at age ten. Varicocele occurs when the testicular veins are anomalously dilated, causing the blood to stagnate in proximity to one or both testicles.

A Story of Tenderness and Trust

Silvia is a dear friend, and her son Bernardo is eight years old. One evening in December, when I stop by her house to exchange Christmas gifts, she asks me in passing if I have time to take a look at her son. She tells me that she thinks his weenie is having trouble uncovering itself and remaining uncovered, and her concerns are accentuated by the fact that Giacomo, her husband, was circumcised as a baby. Her mother-in-law has always been reluctant to reveal the reason for that operation and her husband doesn't remember. In his house no one mentions the genitals; even colloquially using words like "dick" and "pussy" are strictly off-limits. From a brief search on the internet, Silvia thinks her son might suffer from frenulum breve. Bernardo doesn't want to hear about it, however, he refuses to be examined.

I ask him if I can look at him from a distance without touching anything, at least to get an idea, but he won't listen and hides behind the couch, screaming. Giacomo and Silvia apologize, and I have no choice but to leave him be: never force a child to be examined. I tell Bernardo that I won't examine him until he wants me to, indulging in a doctor's little white lie. It isn't possible to wait forever, of course, partly because if there's a real problem operating quickly is fundamental. I ask Silvia to take a photo or make a brief video while Bernardo is showering.

Several days later I receive a message from her on Whatsapp, from which it emerges that the diagnosis is not frenulum breve, but rather phimosis, as I suspected from the story of his father's circumcision.

A month later Bernardo is in the hospital, clinging tightly to the stuffed animal his grandfather gave him.

We joke a little bit and I repeat that there's no need for an examination but that, if he lets himself fall asleep, he'll wake up with a brand-new weenie.

At dinner at Giacomo and Silvia's six months later, he comes over and whispers in my ear: "Thanks for my super weenie." I'm even happier than he is.

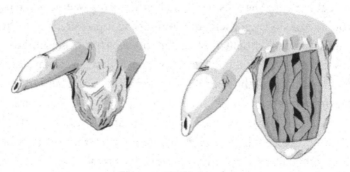

Figure n. 13—Varicocele

To understand the nature of this condition, it's worth remembering that the testicles are appendages external to the human body, because optimal spermatogenesis—sperm production—usually requires a temperature lower than that of the body. A vein, for its part, is defined as varicose when it doesn't function correctly, preventing the blood from circulating fluidly (think of varicose veins in the legs, which dilate to the point of being visible to the naked eye).

Varicocele appears 95% of the time in the left-hand testicle for reasons of anatomy: on the left the spermatic vein reaches the renal vein at a 90-degree angle, while on the right the angle is more acute and thus easier to reach. What's created is a sort of malfunction in the funicular that carries blood from the testicles to the body.

Varicocele occurs when a vein becomes varicose near a testicle. The stagnation of blood provokes an increase in temperature, which over time can create chronic harm and even lead to fertility problems. Note, however, that infertility is not a parallel condition to the appearance of varicocele: there are frequent cases of young men between 18–20 with varicocele who are also fertile.

The pathology is quite common—an average of 15–20% of boys suffer from it—though the seriousness of the phenomenon can vary. The conditions that merit clinical attention are those termed "third degree," or visible to the naked eye (a swelling similar to a ball of yarn can be seen), and identifiable via examination by a specialized doctor, who can detect the existence of stagnancy or reflux even by touch. Usually the discomfort or pain caused by varicocele is amplified after physical strain, such as during sports. So pay attention to the warning signs: if after a training session, a game or a swim meet your child complains of pain, don't ignore it, have it looked at.

The treatment for serious cases of varicocele is essentially surgical and should be done before age twenty. I don't recommend waiting any longer, because it isn't possible to identify beforehand which cases of varicocele might lead to infertility.

The decision on how to proceed must also be made keeping in mind the size of the testicle concerned. The vein responsible for raising the temperature, in fact, can even create a reduction in the volume of the testicle, which is then prevented from developing correctly. Varicocele affects roughly 15% of children, but the decision to proceed or not with the operation varies according to the pain and seriousness of the pathology. An operation is called for only if the varicocele is defined as third degree, on a clinical scale that goes from 1 (slight) to 3 (serious).

The operation itself is rather simple and lasts an average of 15–20 minutes. It consists of a small incision at groin level to connect the veins and thus eliminate the reflux, direct cause of the rise in temperature around the testicle.

Radiological interventions are also a possibility. By using a probe and exploiting the circulatory system, we reach the spermatic veins and close them with sclerotizing substances. But these are invasive procedures that require more time and have an 8% relapse rate, far higher than the 1% associated with the traditional surgical technique.

Once the more traditional operation has been performed, it's best for the patient to take it easy for about a week and avoid any sporting activities for a month. After which life can continue in good health.

Now that the occasion of the draft physical, ideal for the mass screening of young men, has disappeared, it is everyone's responsibility to find other paths to keep tabs on the health of the genital organs. The risk, in fact, is that, in the absence of that unique opportunity to diagnose and treat a whole series of solely male pathologies in a timely manner, intervention may come too late.

Hydrocele

Hydrocele is similar to varicocele in terms of their assonance and the area impacted, but not in what it entails. It consists in the spillage of a serous liquid between the scrotal sac and the testicle, which thus swells suddenly, sometimes even becoming a purplish color, causing an inflammation or even an infection. In adolescents and adults it can appear following operations to treat varicocele, or in correlation with traumas or other pathologies. In children it usually occurs due to a lack of closure of the communication channel between the abdomen and scrotum during fetal development, an opening that leads to the collection of this fluid. Describing it this way makes it seem very complex and a little worrying, but it's very rare (affecting less than 1% of children). It's considered normal up to eighteen months, a window of time in which it can go away on its own, but after which it's necessary to intervene. The swelling is often less visible in the morning and more so at the end of the day.

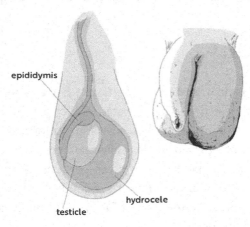

Figure n. 14—Hydrocele

Another cause of hydrocele is what's known as **newborn genital crisis**. This definition, which tends to generate excessive alarm mainly due to the word "crisis," is simply a collection of phenomena typical of the first days of life due to an elevated quantity of hormones, which through the placenta are passed from mother to son or daughter (in fact it affects both males and females). It's a condition without risks, which resolves itself within a few weeks. During this period the genitals appear swollen, as do the breasts. We often see transitory hydroceles which then disappear; it takes the child time to assimilate this excess of hormones.

A hydrocele is generally treated with antibiotics that help reabsorb the liquid. If it persists, it's necessary to undergo surgery, which consists of extracting the testicle to clean it and then reposition it in its proper place. Recovery time is around thirty days.

For the majority of the pathologies that we've discussed up to this point there's no particular prevention we can undertake, given that we're dealing with congenital conditions. Only timely checkups will permit an early diagnosis, thanks to which generally manageable and non-invasive solutions can be adopted.

EMERGENCIES

This section is dedicated to accidents, to what we can't predict and inevitably catches us unprepared. We can have a perfect penis, clean and in order, but anything, unfortunately, can happen. Traumas in and of themselves are certainly possible, but they're less frequent than we fear, particularly in smaller children. In case of an accident, it's a good idea to apply ice immediately and go to the nearest ER to verify the seriousness of the damage done.

Then there's what's called **testicular torsion**, one of the most common emergencies. It's a clinical condition in which the time factor is crucial. In fact it needs to be resolved within six-to-twelve hours of its appearance to avoid irreversible damage.

The Saving Power of Light

The problems with a hydrocele arise during diagnosis, because it isn't easy to distinguish it from an inguinal hernia. On a single day of visits, in fact, I've observed the same symptoms in multiple patients that concealed different pathologies.

Stefano comes to see me at the clinic, he's seven years old and for several days he's had an extremely swollen testicle. I take a flashlight and shine it at it from behind: I notice a transparency at the light's passage. Then I push the testicle toward the groin, to see whether it disappears or shrinks, but nothing happens. I tell Stefano's mother that he clearly has a hydrocele, but that I'll ask for an ultrasound to be sure. If the testicle had shrunken or there hadn't been that transparency, I would've said inguinal hernia, but the question is simpler. Stefano isn't interested in our conversation or his voluminous testicle. He waits for the examination to finish and then asks for the soccer cards his mother had promised him.

Just two hours earlier I examined Carlo, eleven, who had the same problem as Stefano, with the sole difference that his swelling had been there for a year. No one had noticed because Carlo wouldn't let his mom and dad see him naked, demonstrating a perhaps excessive embarrassment. One evening his mother had noticed an anomalous swelling under his pajama bottoms, and even after imploring him, Carlo wouldn't let her see. So they had reached a compromise: I would examine him, on the condition that his mother keep her back turned for the entire visit. The flashlight's response was different than in Stefano's case.

To distinguish a hydrocele from a hernia, even before the results of the ultrasound, this simple experiment is often sufficient. If light shines through, it's a hydrocele, otherwise we're looking at a hernia.

An inguinal hernia is generated when a part of the intestine "protrudes," a complicated verb to say that it sticks out in an anomalous way, making its way into the inguinal canal and ending up on the testicle. It's resolved surgically by putting the intestine back in its place and then inserting a small net, to prevent the situation from recurring in the future.

The situation generally comes about at night. The child is awakened by a sudden and violent spasm of the testicle, which can extend to the abdomen. The pain can be so intense that it generates fits of nausea and vomiting. The trigger is the torsion of the spermatic cord—the structure that contains the vessels that bathe the testicle—which, as it twists, causes an ischemia of the testicle itself, which appears swollen, while the external scrotum takes on a bluish color.

In these situations it's best to go straight to the closest ER—possibly one with a pediatric specialty—that can immediately operate on the child. Speed is important, because if within six hours of the appearance of the symptoms the chances of saving the testicle are between 80–100%, after twelve hours they're near zero. Often it's precisely the cessation of pain that signals that the testicle is dead. In this case, removal is absolutely necessary.

A factor that entails an added complication lies in the difficulty of diagnosis. Testicular torsion, in fact, can be confused with **rotation of the testicular appendage** (hydatid of Morgagni) or **acute epididymitis** (the inflammation of the epididymis that often occurs in response to an infection). Doubts are generally dispelled with specific exams, but if even a testicular Doppler ultrasound is unable to establish a clear diagnosis, exploratory surgery becomes necessary.

In the case of rotation, the surgeon proceeds with a counter-torsion of the testicle with one hand and sets it with three stitches. The other testicle is then set in the same manner, given that those who develop a torsion in one of the two are generally subject to doing so in the second as well.

The Old "Zipper Caught on the Foreskin"

It's ten minutes to six on a July afternoon and I'm about to finish my shift. For months I've been living in London, where I'm doing the last year of my specialization at King's College. Every day at six I get changed, walk to the station which is three minutes away, take the train to Victoria Station, and in exactly fifteen minutes I'm home. My roommate, a nice Englishman of Indian origins, has organized a traditional Indian dinner which is sure to be excellent.

Just as I'm about to set off toward the changing room my beeper goes off. I stop at the first telephone I find (it's the year 2000 and cellphones still aren't that common) and I call the ER. They ask me to come down quickly and from the stairwell I can already hear a young patient's screams.

His name is Peter, he's six years old, and they tell me he's been screaming like a banshee ever since he stepped foot in the clinic. He's wearing a t-shirt and from the waist down he's completely naked, except for a shred of pants stuck to his penis. When I get closer I realize that in reality it's only the zipper, which the mother Jennifer didn't try to force but actually lightened by cutting off the jeans around it. They rushed to the ER with the zipper attached to the foreskin. His mother, desperate, explains that it's her fault.

She tells me sobbing: "Peter is slow, even when he has to go pee, and seeing as we had to go out for dinner I took him to the bathroom and pulled his pants down, had him go and then firmly pulled the zipper up." Peter continues to cry inconsolably. I reassure the mother and focus on the child, telling him that we'll resolve the problem in a minute. First I apply an anesthetic cream to the foreskin and the zipper: in just a few minutes it takes effect, Peter is calmer. I, on the contrary, am quite nervous, but resonating in my head is what my dad Paolo always told me: never let a patient see you hesitant. I ask for a lubricant and spread it practically everywhere: the more slippery it is, the better.

There's only one thing left to do. Delicately but firmly I remove the zipper. Peter's foreskin bleeds a little, but the wound is very small and will heal on its own. All in all, nothing serious. Jennifer and Peter are ready to go home and I run to the station, anticipating my chicken tikka masala. As soon as I enter the building I smell a delicious little aroma of spices and when I put my key in the lock and open the door, the whole gang crowded around the table turns toward me. From their guilty looks I realize that there's nothing left. I defrost a frozen pizza and explain why I'm late. A few days later, I get an Indian dinner in consolation.

It was the first time I was faced with a penis caught in a zipper, but certainly not the last. In fact it's a common accident, especially among children. The important thing is not to panic and act calmly but immediately. Zippers are devious and the only way to get free of them is with a firm tug. But careful, better to leave it to a professional. Be like Jennifer and Peter, go straight to the ER to avoid acting like a di . . . mwit.

If you've undergone an operation like this at a young age—before eighteen—I always recommend getting a fertility screening. If there's an anomaly in the spermiogram, the sooner you act, the better your chances of solving the problem.

Another emergency situation is **paraphimosis**. Unlike phimosis, it occurs when the foreskin, after sliding up the shaft, struggles to reposition itself. So there could be a partial or total sliding of the foreskin, which is open at the glans, and that the foreskin, once it retracts, is no longer able to return to its starting position, thus constricting the glans.

It's important to intervene quickly for the manual repositioning of the foreskin, even recurring to the assistance of local anesthetics. You want to avoid the risk of the situation degenerating toward necrosis, when the foreskin, squeezing the base of the glans, stops the flow of blood to the tip of the penis. Only rarely is surgery necessary, which consists of an incision in the foreskin to allow the skin to resume sliding and cover the glans. Later, circumcision is recommended.

Lastly, I always remind people that before letting the child into the bath it's important to check the water temperature. It seems like a no-brainer, but at the ER burns of the genital area caused by excessively hot water are more frequent than you might think.

We want to soothe adults' anxiety and for this reason we've covered all possible events. But it's important to keep in mind that the likelihood of the pathologies described here is, on average, low: I hope that my explanation helps to dispel your doubts and provide serenity.

Congenital pathologies aside, in childhood problems are generally not serious. The good stuff (so to speak) comes in the following chapters.

2

THE ADOLESCENT PENIS

"Why don't you mind your own business?"

In the individual, adolescence is the stage of evolutionary passage between childhood and adulthood, a transition that occurs on average in the interval between twelve-thirteen and eighteen years of age. Here we've decided to avoid characterizing the various phases of life with age ranges, since the passage from one to another is extremely subjective. Adolescence could begin at eleven, just as it could begin at fifteen; the important thing is knowing how to identify when it's beginning.

This, then, is a period of life characterized by profound changes, in the body but also in the mind. The penis goes through a phase of accelerated growth due to the increased activity of the pituitary gland, which then provokes a greater dynamism in the suprarenal glands, the thyroid and the testicles. At the end of the process, we are looking at a physically adult individual.

The dad in me would begin this chapter by discussing the frustration and the concern that nag parents when their children enter this delicate developmental phase. But I want the focus to be on the kids. On the ones who see their body change and become an entity equipped with its own dynamics, with which they have to learn to grapple in the space of a few months or, at most, in a couple of years. The transition process is naturally a long one and this is true for everyone: adults mustn't think they can abdicate from their role of supervision and guidance overnight, but they must begin to step back. Resigning themselves, for example, to the fact that they'll no longer see their children walking around the house naked.

UPKEEP

This phase of life is dedicated to discovery and experimentation. Hey, there's a dick down there! It's active, awake. It gets hard for no reason precisely to remind us that it's there, it exists.

Between the age of twelve and sixteen the penis goes through a phase of intense development, consistent with the transformations that affect the rest of the body. At the beginning of puberty the scrotum and testicles grow larger, while at the base of the shaft appears the first pubic hair, though it's still sparse. Later, the penis takes on a more intense coloration, the glans its classic conformation, and the scrotum grows further. The genitals begin to resemble those of an adult, in both size and shape. The features acquired by the age of eighteen-twenty are those that the individual will have as a mature adult, bringing an end to this whirlwind of changes.

The leitmotiv of this phase is "harmony." The organism as a whole evolves in a proportionate and balanced way toward its adult forms. I know very well that at first the explosion won't seem too harmonious: some kids shoot up in height in just a few months, start sprouting hair on what's still a child's face, or find themselves with a different voice from one day to the next. Don't despair: as in any explosion, after the blast everything will find its proper place.

Being Precocious

Juri is seven years old. He's one of the tallest kids in his class, a few kilos overweight, and he even has a little hair on his face and body. His Uncle Ascanio tells me about it, worried because, ever since last vacation, whenever they get together with his brother's family, Juri creates problems with his two sons, Alberto and Andrea, nine and seven, with whom he'd always gotten along fine.

"I mean, doctor, they always end up fighting, they actually hit one another. Juri has had problems at school too. My brother jokes about it, he says that he was like this as a kid too. I'm worried, this isn't just rowdiness. If something isn't done, he risks becoming a bully."

I'm certainly aware of how important it is to recognize bullying quickly, especially after my son Michele was a victim of it several years ago. He talked to us about it right away and we got through it, thanks in part to the help of teachers who were very well prepared on the subject. Today he's moved past it and gained confidence in himself: bullying him isn't so easy anymore, partly because he's taken up boxing.

Ascanio's story makes me suspect that something else is going on. I ask a few more questions about the physical traits of this child, with a more-than-above-average height and pronounced body hair at an early age. I ask Ascanio to talk to his brother to investigate the matter further.

"From what you've told me it could be a case of precocious

puberty—quite rare in males and, consequently, little talked about—that can be caused by a precocious activation of the hypothalamus-hypophysis-testicles system, but which can sometimes be a symptom of serious genetic diseases or cancer."

I also tell him to insist that Juri's father take him to an endocrinologist for an evaluation. But he also needs to take a step back on the bullying question, which causes his brother to clam up. If there's a problem, it's necessary to deal with it quickly and without jumping to conclusions.

The endocrinologist confirms a diagnosis of early puberty and prescribes a series of tests, the outcome of which requires hormone therapy. After two months of the therapy, Juri is back to being a tranquil "child" of seven, with all due respect to his uncle and cousins.

You might think that diagnosing early puberty is simple, that it suffices to observe a six-year-old girl developing breasts or a seven-year-old boy with underarm hair. But it's actually far more complicated.

Puberty is considered "precocious" when it begins in females before eight and in males before nine. The estimates vary, but the statistics say that it affects roughly one in five thousand children, predominantly females.

There are two types. The most common is central precocious puberty, when the brain begins the normal process of puberty—setting off the release of various hormones—just earlier. In most cases there's no particular reason. Then there's peripheral precocious puberty, which is rarer. It usually develops when there's an excess production of sexual hormones due to a cyst or tumor, so it's necessary to investigate further.

There are different paths for diagnosing early puberty. It usually begins with a physical exam to evaluate the changes in the body. An analysis of family history is equally important, to find out whether there have already been other cases (in fact we can say that Juri's father, who was "like this" as a kid, suffered from precocious puberty, though not to the extent of his son).

Next are blood tests to check the child's hormonal and thyroid levels, and an x-ray, usually of the hand or the wrist, to check bone age: this is an accurate way to see how quickly the growth process is proceeding and which problems could arise in the future.

An MRI of the brain can also exclude medical problems at the root of precocious puberty, such as cancer. This is done only in extreme cases, as in children under six or with other symptoms. The opposite condition also exists—delayed puberty. In this case we find an absence of development of the testicles by the age of fourteen, often accompanied by a lack of underarm and pubic hair. The most frequent cause is a constitutional or growth delay, or more rarely a pathological condition known as hypogonadism, in which the testicles don't produce sufficient levels of hormones. For the diagnosis the same tests are prescribed as for suspected precocious puberty. In rare cases recourse is made to a testosterone-based hormone therapy, but most times the situation is simply monitored without any specific treatment.

Ideally all boys would undergo an andrological exam concurrent with adolescence or the beginning of sexual activity. It's rather unlikely, in fact, for a family doctor to check a teenage boy's genitals except in the presence of specific illnesses or visible anomalies; yet the age of kids' first sexual experiences tends to be around fifteen-sixteen.

Beyond the medical side of things, a checkup by a specialist could also facilitate a resolution of the "size problem." Boys have a partly distorted vision of the question: if you asked them what the normal size of a penis should be, they would answer "around 18 centimeters," while adapting the perception of their own body to this number. A urologist could set them straight in a few seconds.

The widespread availability of pornographic images that suggest completely abnormal standards doesn't help, and actually represents a cause of stress. The word of a doctor can sometimes placate anxieties that are difficult to express out loud: sex in pornography doesn't correspond to the norm, even in the most extreme cases.

Now dads might object that we've all made use of pornography, even before internet (we all remember the magazines purchased collectively, and the shame felt by the one who had to ask the guy at the newsstand). And in fact I'm not saying that it should be prohibited, kids would look at it anyway. The question is when. It needs to happen at the appropriate moment, when they're able to look critically at what they see and not be overwhelmed. The implications are endless and concern our deepest emotional spheres.

The correct transmission of information becomes a tool for overcoming borderline and potentially critical situations. For example, the timing in which the question of penis size is posed is often wrong, which is also the reason it risks degenerating. At twelve or thirteen it's difficult to provide exact numbers: only the indicator of "harmony," in fact, can give an indication. Height and build, as we've said, have their importance. We should wait until at least sixteen-eighteen years of age—the end of the developmental phase—before making a precise evaluation.

This chronic and needless preoccupation for a presumed flaw attributed to one's body is called **dysmorphophobia**, a word that, if it were easier to write and articulate, would certainly match the popularity of the term "resilience" because it perfectly represents a widespread feeling among adolescents. With the publication of my studies on penis size, my life has changed. For years I was invited to conferences around the world and my clinic was invaded by thousands of kids who wanted a longer penis. Yet their penis was actually almost always in the norm. In 70% of cases, the people who came to me finally found peace of mind.

People with a distorted view of their own body—sufferers of dysmorphophobia—are at serious risk of perennial dissatisfaction. Rather than a surgical solution, my advice in these cases is a consult of a psycho-sexual nature. In medical terms at least, size is entirely secondary.

Continuing to discuss the difference between the expectations of the outside world and the concrete nature of our physicality, we are now going to look at **gender dysphoria**.

We've decided to make this section a bit less playful, because in order to bring out its complexity it's necessary to use a precise vocabulary that corresponds with the delicate feelings and sensations of the human mind. If the penis is an organ composed of multiple and varying equilibria, we must always remember that it's only one piece of that complicated puzzle that is the individual.

The many studies and investigations of the relation between sexuality, biological sex and gender have created a variegated and complex theoretical and clinical picture, as well as a terminology whose definitions still remain a terrain for debate and interpretation. To approach gender dysphoria, or that feeling of clinical suffering and inadequacy with respect to the gender assigned at birth, it's important to make certain linguistic distinctions.

Sex identifies the individual as "male" or "female" based on **sexual characteristics** existing from birth. These characteristics are classified as **primary** (chromosomes, morphology of the genitals, gonads and hormonal picture) or **secondary** (hair distribution and density, breast development, characteristics of muscular development). Sex is thus the result of many interactions, which end up conditioning the physiology of the body and the brain.

The **concept of gender,** on the other hand, lies outside of the purely biological field and refers to factors and influences with cultural, social and psychological characteristics. Different cultures can have different parameters of masculinity or femininity; gender identity is simply a question of identifying oneself or not, of how you perceive yourself, vis-à-vis these parameters.

Particularly in recent years the traditional binarism between male and female has frequently been disputed, symptomatic of the fact that our society is slowly beginning to move forward.

Many people identify only partly or temporarily with the man-woman dichotomy, and those who present or identify themselves with a gender that doesn't conform to their biological sex are generally referred to as **transgender.** In this realm the Italian language has its limits: in Anglophone and Germanic languages, culturally ahead of us in this area, a lack of identification with the canonical genders corresponds to the use of the pronoun "They," as an alternative to "She" and "He." The international terminology is thus more fitting because it has abandoned many of the stereotypes that create excessively constrictive cages for individual identity.

The **sexual and emotional orientation** of transgender people is independent of their identifying themselves or not in one of the two genders: sexual and emotional attraction toward people of the same sex (homosexuality), the opposite sex (heterosexuality) or both sexes (bisexuality) is in fact not connected to feeling oneself to be male or female. The sense of estrangement from one's own body is usually reflected in behaviors and attitudes, and is manifested in different ways according to age and biological sex.

During childhood kids can express discomfort and unhappiness with their sex in more or less explicit ways, with strong emotional involvement and a desire to belong to the opposite sex. But this doesn't mean that boys who play with Barbies or girls who play with cars automatically suffer from gender dysphoria.

In adolescence, the intensity of the desire to belong to the opposite sex can become even stronger, interfering with the individual's personal activities and social relations. If this is experienced in solitude or, worse still, in an oppressive atmosphere due to external factors, it can lead to depression and self-isolation.

Adolescence is a period of crucial importance for the realization of personal identity. With growth comes an increase in awareness and the ability to perceive our social and cultural environment, and a consequent increase in doubts, uncertainties and anxieties. But this mustn't lead to a closure toward the outside. One of the greatest risks associated with gender dysphoria is constituted by the progressive social isolation brought on by this distress. This isolation can be induced by the scorn of one's peers for certain "quirky" behaviors and lead to a dangerous lowering of self-esteem. It's important to find someone with whom to speak freely, a friend or, more often, an external professional figure who assists in understanding the bigger picture. To this end there are also free counseling services at school, which should certainly be taken into consideration.

The process of comprehending and accepting your own image is also defined as "body mentalization" and represents the ability to make the way we appear coherent with our own inner values.

Gender dysphoria is manifested as the desire to free ourselves of our primary or secondary sexual characteristics, to be treated as members of the opposite or of neither gender, to acquire a more fluid identity. In Italy, **the National Observatory of Gender Identity (ONIG)** is the point of reference for all those who think or are certain that they don't identify with their biological sex, providing information and orientation and offering specialized assistance.

In medical terms, however, it's indispensable to begin a path involving multiple specialists, aimed first and foremost at understanding whether we're looking at a transitory or a definitive choice. Obviously timing has its importance, because waiting and postponing can entail negative psychological and physical consequences for those wishing to undertakes this type of transition.

Reviewing my own clinical experience, I'd say that twenty years ago it was largely men who decided to follow this road. They first went through an intermediate phase, disguising themselves in some way, before deciding on a sex change as adults, around the age of thirty-five, forty, even fifty. Today, however, there are processes of accompaniment and hormone therapies that make it easier for boys and girls—while they're still in the developmental phase—to modify their secondary sexual characteristics. With our more advanced surgical capabilities, we can achieve extremely satisfying results that can truly improve people's lives.

Now let's look at the surgical operation for changing gender. The truth of the matter is that Italian law doesn't allow this for minors, so it would be more correct to discuss this topic in the chapter on adulthood. But we want to introduce it here to allow adolescents who are experiencing this difficult condition to see a potential way out and familiarize themselves with this possibility.

The path to get there is very long and calls for certain obligatory steps: first psychological support, then hormone therapy accompanied by an endocrinologist, and finally a legal procedure with lawyers to enact the definitive change of sex at the bureaucratic level. Surgery is merely the final part, and it isn't even obligatory.

When you decide to go down this road, one of the difficulties you face is the cost of the transition. I'd like to underline that, since October 1, 2020, the cost of hormone therapy is covered by the National Health Service and that, even if you decide to have the operation in the future, it's possible to put yourself on a waiting list at public hospitals. Cost needn't be a cause of fear.

Concretely, the **operation for male-to-female transition (MTF)** consists in two stages. The first, "destructive" stage eliminates the penis—leaving a small portion of it that will later serve to form the clitoris, thus preserving sensitivity and nerve stimulations—and removes the testicles. The second, "reconstructive" stage creates the vagina with skin from the scrotum.

After the operation, the patient must use dilators for several months, which serve to create a near-natural vaginal space, because over time this passage tends to heal and close up. Those who have undergone this type of operation say that they're able to experience a satisfying sexual life, though here we are entering a territories quite difficult to analyze or comment on.

In an **operation for female-to-male transition (FTM)** the end result is more complicated to achieve, because the penis, in order to achieve erection, exploits a hydraulic mechanism that has to be built—and it's always easier to destroy than it is to create, as any builder will tell you, but the strictly surgical side is simpler. The process calls for the creation of strips of skin and the construction of a sleeve—it resembles a penis more in appearance than in structure—which, however, lacks functionality since it can't ejaculate. A penile prosthesis is then inserted to enable the sexual act and recreate the system of valves and tie-beams.

The discovery of pleasure certainly doesn't occur during puberty—as children we explore our genitals almost casually, instinctively—but during puberty it takes hold in a significant way. And **masturbation** has a starring role. With the erotic impulse due to hormones, in fact, boys and girls practice it naturally. The search for pleasure is a fundamental right of men and women.

One of the most entertaining books I've ever read on the subject is Philip Roth's *Portnoy's Complaint*. Alex Portnoy's long monologue on his therapist's couch brings to light his obsessions with masturbation, to which he dedicates an entire chapter. "Whacking Off," in fact, begins like this:

"Then came adolescence—half my waking life spent locked behind the bathroom door, firing my wad down the toilet bowl, or into the soiled clothes in the laundry hamper, or *splat*, up against the medicine-chest mirror, before which I stood in my dropped drawers so I could see how it looked coming out. [. . .] Through a world of matted handkerchiefs and crumpled Kleenex and stained pajamas, I moved my raw and swollen penis, perpetually in dread that my loathsomeness would be discovered by someone stealing upon me just as I was in the frenzy of dropping my load. Nevertheless, I was wholly incapable of keeping my paws from my dong once it started the climb up my belly. In the middle of a class I would raise a hand to be excused, rush down the corridor to the lavatory, and with ten or fifteen savage strokes, beat off standing up into a urinal. At the Saturday afternoon movie I would leave my friends to go off to the candy machine—and wind up in a distant balcony seat, squirting my seed into the empty wrapper from a Mounds bar."

Flicking the bean, beating the meat, jacking off, jerking it, knocking one out, playing solitaire, polishing the pearl, spanking the monkey. What is male masturbation?

The most precise definition is certainly the one that speaks of autoeroticism, a term whose frigidity manages to calm even the most hot-blooded spirits. To underline its crudest (and slightly cruel) side, the English use "to choke the chicken," while the Germans opt for the more pragmatic *Fünf gegen einen*, "five-on-one." I don't imagine that a book like this is revealing anything that you don't already know, but seeing as by now we're among friends, we might as well confront the topic.

In 1994 Jocelyn Elders, a pediatrician and President Bill Clinton's Surgeon General, was forced to resign just hours after publicly declaring that masturbation ought to be taught in public schools.

Even today such a statement arouses at best laughter, at worst aversion.

As Roth recounts, masturbation is too often associated with guilt and the fear of being discovered. After all, the term "masturbation," from the Latin *manus*, "hand", and *stuprare*, "to contaminate," seems to infer something dirty, though it hasn't always been this way. In Egyptian civilization, it referred to the genesis of life, or the god Artum, who by spreading his seed on the earth gave life to the first living beings.

Grafted onto such activity, then, is an endless series of cultural and religious conditionings, generally of the derogatory sort. The arguments usually derive from the conception, now almost a thing of the past, that sex serves only for procreation and thus masturbation, which doesn't lead to pregnancy, is an impure act. Centuries ago people believed that the quantity of sperm in a man was limited, and thus wasting it was a genuine sin. Naturally this is false.

Even the rumor about blindness has, fortunately, returned to being just that. The reason it's so widespread must be linked to Samuel Tissot, an 18th-century Swiss doctor who argued that in ejaculation zinc, an element that protected the eye from light, was expelled from the human body, thus jeopardizing our sight. Only in the early 20th century, with the birth of modern sexology and thanks to the work of Alfred Kinsey—about whose story a film has even been made, with his last name as the title—have we returned to a more balanced and positive vision.

One of the potential benefits of this practice is that through masturbation we're able to explore our sexuality without the inopportune involvement of another person, independently discovering what we like and what we don't. We can thus prepare ourselves for a dialogue with a future partner. For science it's a wholly natural act, which actually protects the urogenital system—particularly the prostate—and reinforces the immune system and the individual's emotional and psychological health. It must also be said that, for adolescents, masturbation is a far safer sexual outlet than unsafe intercourse, with its ramifications of sexually-transmitted diseases, undesired pregnancies and emotional implications. Plus masturbation generates self-esteem and a momentary sense of relief and relaxation—but you probably didn't need a doctor to figure that out.

Naturally it shouldn't become an obsession or a means for avoiding relations with others, as in Portnoy's case: this would be a warning sign of a situation of discomfort that should be faced with the help of a specialist. At the risk of sounding repetitive, I always recommend talking about it openly, rather than letting it become a problem.

During adolescence, the penis hardens even without particular stimuli. I'm referring to **nocturnal erections,** which we notice upon waking: they occur in sleep's REM phase—REM stands for Rapid Eye Movement—the one in which we dream. They're completely natural, can even last for a few minutes, and generally pass unobserved. They perform the task of keeping the penis in functioning shape, its tissues active and elastic, and are often accompanied by **emissions,** or releases of sperm—this is why you might wake up with wet underwear. Nothing out of the ordinary—it's the body telling you that everything's in order.

Medical science usually monitors these nocturnal, REM-phase erections via the RigiScan, a device that, using two ring-shaped sensors placed around the penis, makes it possible to register variations in shaft diameter during sleep.

In adulthood, such monitoring helps understand whether a patient complaining of erectile dysfunction has problems of the organic or psychogenic sort. In the former case, he won't get erections at night either. Vice versa, if the nature of the problem is psychogenic, he won't them while awake, due to the psychological control factor (such as performance anxiety), but he will at night.

I'm often asked if it's realistic to speak of **performance anxiety** for an adolescent. The answer is yes. We all remember our first time, our heart racing and the feeling of not being up to the task.

To be precise, however, we need to dig deeper and once again distinguish between erectile dysfunction and what's commonly called "performance anxiety."

Unlike what we're led to believe, erectile dysfunction is not a disease but rather the symptom of a variety of pathologies. Plus a great deal depends on the frequency with which it appears. If we cough a couple of times a week, we certainly don't go to the doctor. In the same way, if the problem occurs sporadically, it should be met with a smile and nothing else. But if it crops up continually, it's better to have some tests run. Problems linked to erection, in fact, are signs of diabetes.

In my experience, erectile dysfunction is a rare pathology in adolescence. Out of a hundred sixteen-to-eighteen-year-old boys who complain of it, ninety-nine of them suffer from erectile dysfunction due to performance anxiety. In these cases, the problem is less that of getting an erection than of maintaining it, and this immediately help to clarify the situation.

The penis, in fact, functions like a hydraulic system and erections occur thanks to a passive mechanism. Unlike a limb, whose movement is commanded by a conscious effort—so that, for example, if I want to raise a glass I have to send an order that corresponds to exercising a force regulated by the release of adrenaline—the penis functions in the opposite way. In order to rise it has to be relaxed, there's no need to intervene with any active impulse.

It's natural that if the mind begins to wonder "Will I be up to the task? Will I be good? It's my first time, I'm scared, will I manage?" the body will induce a charge of adrenaline that blocks the penis and prevents it from doing its work. Contraction is the enemy of erection, unlike what happens with muscles.

When I was twenty-two, after a long and fruitless courtship of a close female friend, one evening—when I'd already lost all hope—she finally looked me in the eye and said: "Why don't the two of us ever go further?"

I was immediately gripped by performance anxiety. I had felt ready for five years, it was all I thought about, and now that the time had come I couldn't do the business. I went home embittered, but the most interesting thing is that several years later, at dinner, she confessed that she had felt awful about it, feeling like she was responsible.

We had experienced something typical of the adolescent years. A boy holds in his performance anxiety and transforms it into monsters that are difficult to kill. The girl, on the other hand, interprets the experience as a refusal and goes into crisis, despairing. From that little misunderstanding comes a huge drama.

Here we enter Patrizia's field: communication. Just as it would have been healthier for us to talk about it, the same is true for everyone, regardless of age or life phase. It's implied that if performance anxiety occurs frequently and becomes an insurmountable obstacle, it's best to seek psychological assistance. Today there are even medications which, from a therapeutic standpoint, can help a great deal. But blindly taking a pill to overcome a single, circumscribed problem could be fatal. From performance anxiety it's easy to develop a dependency, even of a psychological nature.

Paradoxically, it's easier for a specialist to manage a man with an organic erection problem, caused by significant pathologies, than an adolescent who's going through the same situation but in a worse emotional state. In my opinion the question can be overcome with a heavy dose of common sense together with rationality, attention and serenity.

It's also my duty to talk about **contraception.** I know, the word alone is enough to bore you, making you roll your eyes and say "Not again!" But as a urologist, I can say with absolute certainty that a large part of the health of the penis during the sexual age depends on the care we take in contraception. I hope that this is a good enough reason for you not to skip to the next chapter.

In the last twenty years information on the use of contraceptives hasn't changed much, despite the fact that we dispose of a greater quantity of evidence—quantity, of course, doesn't necessarily mean quality. The most recent research indicates that only one of four sexually-active young men between fourteen and eighteen years of age constantly uses a prophy-lactic. And if you ask him why he does so, the answer is "To not risk becoming a dad." This in itself is not a good answer, but it's an answer that shows just how much we underestimate the risks of sexually-transmitted diseases. Only 7 percent of the sample indicate prevention as the reason for using a condom.

To be clear, the **condom** is the only method that offers effec-tive protection against sexually-transmitted diseases, which have nothing to do with an unwanted pregnancy. This is why if we're not in a long-term, monogamous relationship and even if our partner uses a form of contraception such as the pill, it's necessary to use one.

A package of six condoms costs around €8 and can be found at the pharmacy or supermarket or any store selling household and personal hygiene products, usually close to the bandages and disinfectants. Even in vending machines near pharmacies, like the ones that sell coffee.

The fact that they can be found here says a lot about their importance for our health.

To buy them you don't need to have a prescription or have to be of legal age: it's like going to buy yogurt. Even for women, it's useful to have them in case their partner, out of carelessness or distraction, doesn't.

The condom appears as a tubular sheath that conforms to the erect penis. At its tip it has a sort of "little bag," or reser-voir, which serves to contain the ejaculated sperm. It's made typically of latex, though there are versions in polyurethane for those with allergies (if we aren't, our partner might be!).

It's classified as a barrier contraceptive, one, that is, that physically prevents the exchange of fluids.

Size Matters (But Only in One Case)

I leave my children at the oratory entrance and I feel observed. Right there and then I don't pay much attention, but it happens the following days as well.

Every morning a tall, skinny young man with a counselor's t-shirt seems on the verge of speaking to me. Maybe he wants to let me in on one of my son Michele's clownish jokes, or ask me to pay the balance of the tuition fee.

The last day he finds the courage and comes over. His name is Giacomo. With the shiftiness of a drug dealer he asks if we can speak alone in a more private area.

"Hello, I apologize for the approach but I heard Michele say that you treat penises."

I'm a bit surprised. "Yes, sure, I'm a urologist."

"Oh, okay, then it's true?"

"Yes, of course it's true, I even teach courses at the university," I say, thinking that, given his age, Giacomo might be thinking about his post-high school future.

"No, yes, well, I actually need, I think, an examination."

Okay, now it's clear. I give him my card. The way I do so maintains the appearance of some illicit exchange.

He thanks me and walks quickly away. I hear him say to a girl coming toward him: "Yeah, an old friend of my dad's."

A few weeks later, after vacation, I find him in the waiting room. "Please come in."

I look at the forms he's filled out. Giacomo is eighteen and in the notes he writes that he suffers from erectile dysfunction.

"Yeah, well, I think so, I'm not the doctor," he says.

I ask him to tell me in detail what's led him to this conclusion. He takes a deep breath.

"Well, I've tried to have sex three times with my girlfriend. I mean, she's not really my girlfriend, let's say she's a girl I'm going out with. Every time I feel ready and we're about to get there, as soon as I put on the condom my thingy goes soft. As if it didn't want to do it, but I do! I'm scared that if I don't resolve this situation she'll start thinking I think she's ugly."

He's even tried to find information on a blog where users talk about their experiences, but he hasn't succeeded in getting an answer: some recommend supplements, others to take it slowly, and some even made fun of him.

I ask him to get undressed for a routine examination. Giacomo is at his first experience and I'm afraid that anxiety is playing a nasty trick on him. Yet he seems like a calm guy, shy but capable of facing a situation that makes him uncomfortable.

I immediately notice that his penis is already well formed and has reached the size of an adult's.

Truth be told it seems like a penis with an above-average circumference, proportionate to his 1.9-m height. Perhaps now the situation is a little clearer. "Go ahead and get dressed."

"Already? Don't you have to do something?"

"Giacomo, which condoms do you use?"

"I'm not sure, Elisa gave them to me, normal ones."

"I'll give you some new ones, try them out and let me know."

In the afternoon, while I'm with a patient, my cellphone screen lights up.

I did it! I don't know how it happened but you have to tell me where I can get these condoms.

With a brief phone call, I tell him that the condoms I gave him don't have anything magical about them and that he's just the same as a few hours ago. He wasn't using the right size condom, and from now on he'll just need to make sure to find them at the supermarket. The correct size condom is essential to avoid pain and discomfort, but also to avoid losing your erection. Try walking around with shoes that are three sizes too small, your feet will beg for mercy. In addition, the risk that an excessively small condom will break is very high, and this alone is a good reason to choose them with care.

Here is the **guide for the perfect use of the condom:**

1. Choose one that's the right size, to avoid it slipping off during intercourse if it's too big, or constricting the penis if it's too small. For the sake of making the right purchase, we're authorized to equip ourselves with a tailor's measuring tape and measure our erect penis. But careful: we're interested in circumference, not length, because it's condoms' diameter that varies. If you don't have one handy, use yarn or thread and mark the point of conjunction with a marker, then measure that with a ruler.

   The most common condoms are suitable for the majority of penises and have a circumference of roughly 11 cm. But the package states the condoms' diameter: the measure that's easiest to find is 52 mm. To spare you the geometry review, I'll provide you below with the correspondences between circumference and the number on the package, so it's easier for you to get oriented.

   There are also more imaginative condoms: ribbed, fruit flavored, colored, glow in the dark. But these are merely aesthetic differences that don't modify their basic function. Take the necessary time to experiment.

Circumference	Diameter on the package
7–9 cm	47 mm
10–11 cm	49 mm
11–11.5 cm	52 mm
11.5–12 cm	57 mm
12–13 cm	60 mm

2. Don't be embarrassed when you purchase them. Buying condoms should make us proud of protecting ourselves and our partner: so let's get our courage up and view it as an act of caring. And if we just can't manage it, we ask a friend to do it for us.

3. Check the expiration date. Like all perishables, condoms too can expire, because the latex deteriorates and loses elasticity. Expired condoms are great for practicing, on your own, how to put them on: they won't harm the penis, but they're useless in terms of protection.

4. Don't keep them in your wallet or in places where the latex can be altered by heat. Don't keep them in your jeans pocket or the bottom of a backpack either, where a pointed object could perforate them. Pay attention to where you buy them as well: a souvenir condom from your trip to Lochness with "Want to see the monster?" written next to an image of Nessie probably won't be of the greatest quality.

5. Don't ask your partner to have sex without one. It's best to talk about this subject when you're not about to engage in intercourse, because it's a question that can ruin intimacy, generate discomfort, and expose both of you to unjustified risks. Ask yourself, rather,

why you don't want to use it; and the fact that this happens in pornos isn't a good reason.

6. Put it on in the moment prior to penetration, when the penis is already hard. It isn't easy, or recommended, to put it on prior to the erection.

7. Place it on the tip of the penis, taking care to press on the reservoir with two fingers, then unroll it along the erect shaft down to the base. If it unrolls easily, we're unrolling it in the right direction. To make sure it adheres and doesn't have air bubbles, press it against the penis. And be careful not to tear it with your fingernails, teeth or any other object. To open the package don't use scissors, but your fingers.

8. After ejaculation, remove it carefully to avoid spilling the sperm. Protect the contents by making a knot, so no one accidentally comes into contact with it.

9. These instructions are always valid, whether your partner is female or male. Condoms aren't just to prevent conception, and they need to be used in homosexual intercourse as well. No one can be sure they aren't a healthy carrier of a sexually-transmitted disease except after medical testing, repeated over time.

10. Should the condom accidentally break—it's rare but possible, especially if it wasn't put on properly—it's best to take a pregnancy test (usually available next to condoms) and certain screening tests for sexually-transmitted diseases (which can be done in specialized labs or, if you suspect a specific disease, using do-it-yourself kits available at the pharmacy).

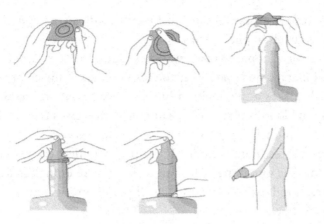

Figure n. 15—How to Put on a Condom

During the 1980s, at the height of the HIV emergency, television and newspapers continually bombarded us with ads about the importance of using condoms. The results were tangible and we witnessed a significant decline in the cases of infection. Then, however, the health emergency ended, the subject was forgotten, and we inevitably lowered our guard.

This gave rise to a whole series of problems. The condom is not just the first line of defense against HIV, which still affects roughly forty million people around the world, but it's also a shield for the whole galaxy of sexually-transmitted pathologies that we'll see in the next section. Even for diseases for which vaccines exist, such as the Papilloma Virus, using a condom remains the only defense. As the recent Covid-19 pandemic has taught us, in the case of viral infections vaccines don't always save us one hundred percent of the time. One in three young men suffer from a genital pathology and, in the absence of screening, almost never know they have it.

December I is World AIDS Day, and the Italian Red Cross sets up gazebos in many Italian cities where you can take a free

HIV test. Alternatively, as I just mentioned, you can purchase one yourself in pharmacies.

It's very simple to take and costs around €25. It consists of a capillary blood sampling; the kit contains a finger pricker, which makes a tiny incision in the index finger. The resulting drop of blood is placed on a white plate that gives the result in fifteen minutes. It's an effective test if you contracted the virus at least three months earlier, but isn't if the infection was more recent. The one thing to be aware of as you're doing the test is to wash and disinfect your hands. If you're positive, further lab tests will be necessary.

Now let's take a look at a subject as simple as it is multifaceted: **pubic hair.** As we've seen, it's only in adolescence that the lower part of the belly is covered with hair, along with the rest of the body. When I was in high school people said that shaving made the penis look longer, but none of us boys had the courage to do it. Paradoxically, the day that a friend of mine came to P.E. completely smooth, everyone started making fun of him for no reason. On this topic medical science and urology have no say in the matter. There are pros and cons, but nothing that says that it's right to do it one way or the other.

More than 25% of those who shave say they've hurt themselves more than once. If you decide to shave, make sure you are very attentive. If you do so with a razor, it must be of the throw-away variety, disinfected with alcohol, and be used exclusively for the genitals. It's best to proceed with the help of shaving cream or genital hygiene product, so as to make everything smoother. The best direction is from below up, from the penis to the belly button. Not all chemical products, such as hair-removal creams, are suitable: some could be too aggressive and cause irritation.

Depilatory wax, on the other hand, is advised against for

extremely sensitive areas, like the testicles. In any case, go to a professional: pulling too hard can cause significant abrasions, and overly hot wax can cause burns.

To conclude the upkeep section, I'd like to introduce a subject that isn't talked about enough.

The statistics tell us that from age fifteen—and up to thirty-five—one of the most insidious forms of **cancer** among young people appears: **testicular cancer.** We still know very little about the causes and risk factors connected to the development of the disease, but the data speak clearly. Just as girls learn to examine their breasts, boys must similarly learn to conduct a **self-examination of the testicles,** crucial for the cancer's early diagnosis. It's important to learn to listen to your body.

Self-examination must take place regularly, generally in the shower, when the skin is the most relaxed, or in front of the mirror, to better observe the areas in question. Place your index and middle fingers behind the testicle and your thumb on the front of it, as if to form a delicate pincer. Move your fingers in a circular motion, allowing you to verify compactness and uniformity. If you feel something that resembles a pebble, a first alarm bell should go off.

Examining both testicles, we might notice certain differences between the two. If one appears hard like a rock, it requires a closer look and this should happen immediately. Often, despite realizing that something is wrong, many adolescent boys wait months before finding the courage to talk about it and organize a visit, wasting precious time. I still remember the case of a boy I visited on August 9 a few years ago. I immediately discovered the testicular tumor, but spent the next two hours arguing with him and his father that I needed to do an ultrasound and operate immediately. But he wouldn't hear of it, the next day he was leaving for Greece.

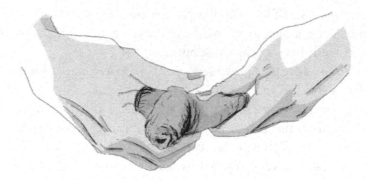

Figure n. 16—Testicular Self-Examination

Thanks to today's therapies, the recovery rate for testicular cancer is 95–99%, even with metastasis. As for all types of cancer, the timing of the diagnosis is fundamental: the sooner you intervene, the less aggressive the protocols that need to be applied.

In the first stage of treatment the classic therapy calls for the complete removal of the testicle in question. To resolve the asymmetry a prosthesis is inserted so that, visually, everything looks right. The healthy testicle will then operate as a "substitute," meaning it works double and compensates for the other's absence.

The radiation therapy and chemotherapy cycles that accompany the surgical phase are now well honed and the state of sterility inevitably induced is merely temporary. In the short term, in fact, there is a return to full fertility. Furthermore, in order to guarantee the possibility of future procreation, when it's necessary to go after the disease clinically, before the beginning of the procedure a fertile sperm sample is frozen. If fertility returns at the end of the protocol, the sperm is eliminated; if not, it can be used.

There is no program of systematic screening for testicular

cancer, and unfortunately the responsibility lies with boys and their families. Roughly 7–8 years ago, the Italian Andrology Society asked me to create a website (www.prevenzioneandrologica.it) which since its launch has reached circa 3–400,000 visits. Users seek help on the most varied problems linked to the male urogenital system.

So the Web can be a good vehicle, even if, as should be clear to you by now, I remain convinced that a conversation focused on sexual education is far more useful. The question of the preparation of the professionals we use certainly needs to be taken into consideration as well, because talking about sexuality requires being precise, exhaustive and unprejudiced.

PATHOLOGIES

We now move to the section dedicated to pathologies. To make things easier, we'll divide the pathologies of the adolescent penis into three categories: **congenital or deriving from childhood; induced by typical adolescent behaviors; or connected to sexuality,** which bursts onto the scene in this period of life.

To the first group belong the conditions we already described in the first chapter, particularly varicocele, hydrocele, phimosis and penile curvature. If untreated, they persist into adolescence: they won't go away by magic.

Varicocele

The period between sixteen and eighteen is when the diagnosis becomes simpler and the symptoms more visible. It's also the best time to proceed to a **potential surgical operation.**

Phimosis

It's generally a congenital pathology that already emerges clearly in childhood. If it appears in adolescence, the related problems could be quite serious: it could be connected to an extremely rare skin disease known as lichen planus, or be a sign of another serious pathology, type-1 diabetes.

In the first case we're dealing with an inflammatory, chronic and progressive skin disease. It's more common in women, which might be why among men it tends to be neglected. In short, **lichen planus** causes the hardening and gradual whitish scarring of the genital tissue. Through growing and successive stages of seriousness, in men it attacks the glans, the meatus and the urethra, even causing stenosis (shrinkage) and blockage. Treatment calls for the applications of salves on the parts affected—useful only to alleviate symptoms—circumcision or the removal of the lesions on the member and its subsequent reconstruction.

With reference to diabetes, phimosis can be a crucially important early warning sign. Even before the classic symptoms—dehydration, excessive thirst, need to urinate often—**type-1 diabetes** can appear, in fact, with penile closure and recurring infections. For this reason, when a non-congenital phimotic state is found in an adolescent, it's necessary to run blood-sugar tests. The treatment will then be calibrated with the stage of the main disease.

Penile Curvature

As we've seen, around twelve years of age the hormones are activated and with them comes an interest in sexuality. We start comparing ourselves to others and become conscious of our own identity, including its physical side.

Adolescence is the best period for addressing and getting over the problem of **penis shape**. The cases of eighteen-year-olds who have never done so and who now, as adults, come to the urologist's office to ask for a consultation, is quite frequent.

The only solution is surgery, preferably on a fully-formed penis. Further delay has no benefits, and could mean denying yourself sexual serenity.

The second group concerns **pathologies caused by adolescent behaviors.** The tensions and turmoil created at the hormonal, emotional and psychological level impact a teenager's body, social life and romantic relations. We seek shelter from our insecurities by doing what everyone does, without thinking of the possible consequences; we're on the lookout for new experiences that until a short while ago we wouldn't have even considered.

The principal pathologies induced by this period of development are linked to alcohol consumption, smoking, and drugs, and their implications for the functioning of the urogenital systems. But these repercussions are actually felt throughout the organism, particularly on the cardiovascular system.

Alcohol Consumption

The medical interpretation is simple and direct: a minimal quantity (one or two glasses) of wine, particularly red, has beneficial effects on both the cardiovascular and neurological systems. The effects are also positive on the mechanism of male erection.

At eighteen, therefore, having a glass at meals is not a problem, but the effects go from positive to negative beyond two glasses. This also occurs in the sexual sphere. In fact alcohol acts as a vasodilator and obstructs the erection mechanism: as the amount ingested increases, you inhibit the pressure in the vessels of the corpora cavernosa and, eventually, the mechanism is blocked.

So it isn't necessary to be an alcoholic to experience its effects; even occasional excessive consumption will suffice. But the constant consumption of high quantities of alcohol can generate erectile dysfunction, which in the long run becomes chronic.

So drinking to shed your inhibitions or overcome shyness and feel lighter when undertaking intercourse is not a good idea.

Alcohol consumption in the delicate period of growth also has serious repercussions on cognitive and physical development. In fact the organism is not yet capable of processing it because it's a complex substance, and you risk blocking or inhibiting the development of the genital system and the hormones that regulate it, such as testosterone.

Smoking

As we know, smoking is harmful for all the functions of our organism, and erection is no exception. In smokers, the first vessel to close up isn't that of the heart, which is relatively large, but rather that of the penis, with a smaller section and therefore at greater risk.

The jeopardizing of cardiovascular functions caused by cigarettes and the like is thus confirmed, indeed, reinforced, when it comes to the male genitals. At any age, even in adolescence, smoking has harmful effects on the sexual sphere, compromising the penis's full functionality and reducing its ability to perform.

Drugs

Drugs—whether of the lighter, natural or the heavier, synthetic variety—are devastating to the organism and, consequently, to the male reproductive system. While they can at first induce positive effects on sexuality—cocaine, for example, gives the impression of resolving premature ejaculation—in the short term and, worse, the long, they set off reactions that severely jeopardize the erection mechanism.

The clinical data and medical research are clear on this point: once we set aside the literary and cinematic mythology, all that remains are the severe consequences on bodily health, the penis included. Feeling uninhibited and spaced out can be dangerous too; when we aren't conscious of what we're doing we adopt risky behaviors which can cause fractures, lesions, or, worse, lead to contracting sexually-transmitted diseases.

The only sensible advice, therefore, is not to use them.

Obesity

Excess weight is one of the worst enemies of correct penile functioning. For an adolescent who has problems with obesity, one of the reasons that can best motivate him to lose weight is the possibility of experiencing a satisfying sexuality.

There are three types of malfunctioning induced by obesity or being overweight.

1. The functioning of the circulatory system, compromised by the excess fat, has repercussions on the **ability to have erections;**
2. The belly's fatty panniculus can end up incorporating the penis, causing a condition that we've already defined as a **buried penis;**

3. Obesity is none other than an accumulation of fat, and thus of estrogens, female hormones: the obese male thus also has a fall in the **quantity of testosterone in circulation,** the first factor in fueling sexual desire.

Piercings

More or less everyone has desired a piercing some point. Genital piercings have a long tradition: ancient civilizations in Africa, Australia and South Asia adopted it and, in some cases, still do to modify the body as a rite of passage. Some call for the perforation of the glans, sometimes the urethra as well, with small bone or metal objects, or the incision of the urethra to make the penis seem larger or give more pleasure to one's partner.

These modifications entail verified, maximal risk profiles. Even the World Health Organization (WHO) has spoken out on the subject, issuing precise and detailed recommendations aiming to discourage as drastically as possible the practices of piercing and tattooing the genitals. They are extremely delicate areas, in which it's easy to unleash severe inflammations or infections.

The WHO's guidelines are stringent: piercings on the penis lead to the creation of a bridge between the urethra—from which urine and semen come out—and the glans, constituting an entryway for infections particularly of the bacterial sort, which in contexts of maximal complication can result in the most serious syndrome that can affect the genitals: Fournier gangrene. This is an extreme situation which requires an emergency operation, and for which there is a 60% chance of death.

VIRAL SEXUALLY-TRANSMITTED DISEASES

We now shift to **sexually-transmitted diseases.** The following is a summary picture of **STDs,** and distinguishes between diseases induced by viral infections and those generated by bacteria. The differentiation concerns both the treatment adopted to fight them and, more generally, implications on quality of life.

AIDS

Today, the best-known sexually-transmitted disease, at least terminologically, is AIDS, or Acquired Immunodeficiency Syndrome. It's caused by two strains of a virus, known as HIV. There is often confusion between the two terms: AIDS is the terminal stage of an infection from HIV.

The acronym stands for Human Immunodeficiency Virus. In 2019 alone, 1.7 million people were found HIV positive around the world; in Italy, there were 3,600 diagnoses, almost ten new infections per day. The number is even higher, however, when we consider how many cases weren't tested or registered: it's these that represent the real danger, because they contribute to the disease's spread.

The diagnosis still occurs too often at an advanced stage, or when the first serious symptoms begin to appear, meaning that the infected person can be a carrier and infect partners without knowing it. HIV can remain latent for many years.

It has been defined "the plague of the 20th century" due to its millions of victims, including the immortal Freddie Mercury, dancer Rudolf Nureyev, artist Keith Haring and the most famous author of science fiction, Isaac Asimov. The HIV viruses are transmitted exclusively during unprotected sexual intercourse with the exchange of bodily fluids—with blood, but even with sperm or vaginal discharge, but not with saliva. Last century the disease was prevalently associated with the worlds of homosexuals—unprotected anal intercourse often causes microcuts and involuntary exchanges of blood—and drug addicts—due to infected syringes shared by different users.

Today, however, we know that HIV is widespread among heterosexuals as well, at a level that's actually superior to that of homosexuals. The disease that derives from it progressively weakens and eventually destroys the immune system. The organism of an AIDS sufferer is defenseless, even against a common cold. At the time of infection you can feel tired or feverish, but nothing more: in the short term it's impossible to suspect infection. This is why prevention and screening are so important.

Thanks to scientific progress, today HIV positivity is no longer a death sentence. Magic Johnson, one of the NBA's greatest all-time players, announced that he was HIV positive in 1991, yet thanks to medicine he continues to live a normal life and his activism in favor of HIV prevention is stronger than ever. Available therapies call for the use of a combination of antivirals capable of preventing the virus's replication in the organism.

The overall effectiveness of the treatment protocols has grown significantly over time, such that today someone with HIV has a survival rate and quality of life comparable to those who haven't contracted the viruses. But it must still be remembered that HIV continues to reside in the cells of the immune system, and that at present a complete cure doesn't exist. A certain continuity is necessary for the treatment to keep the virus at bay.

To eliminate the stigma to which people affected by HIV are still subjected today, it's important to remember that those who are undergoing treatment, those who know they are HIV positive and are fighting it with drugs, don't transmit the virus—U=U: when HIV is no longer detected in the blood following treatment **(Undetectable)**, it is no longer transmittable **(Untransmittable)**.

AIDS is slowly and constantly diminishing, but it's important not to lower our guard. In order to prevent infection, use condoms regularly and correctly. More information on HIV can be found at www.uniticontrolaids.it, on the website of the Ministry of Health, which also has a dedicated toll-free number (www.salute.gov.it/portale/hiv), and at www.anlaidsonlus.it (National Association for the Fight Against AIDS).

Papilloma Virus

A second pathology quite common in young people is HPV (Human Papilloma Virus), known as papilloma. The virus, generally transmitted by the man, is only diagnosed in 10% of patients because the infection it induces is often asymptomatic, produces no visible alterations and goes away on its own.

The dangerousness of HPV lies in the tumoral forms that can arise due to the infection: in women it attacks the uterine neck, in men the penis. Moreover, if it is prolonged over time it can cause diseases of the skin and mucous in the uterine cervix, the larynx, the penis and the anus. HPV can appear with several growths, often called rooster combs due to their features, or with the appearance of warts that cause irritation or itching.

The majority of these types of lesions heal on their own, but sometimes a lack of treatment paves the way for carcinogenic forms. It all depends on the serotype of the virus you come into contact with and the lesions that develop. There are one hundred and twenty types of HPV, but two in particular (HPV

16 and HPV 18) are the principal culprits for the most serious forms.

In cases in which healing doesn't occur spontaneously, warts and rooster combs can be treated with antiviral creams, generally quite effective.

Over the course of a lifetime eight out of ten people come into contact with one of these HPV viruses and infection prevalently occurs via intercourse. But it's the fact that it's prevalently asymptomatic that makes it treacherous. Those who develop its visible symptoms, such as warts or rooster combs, are actually the ones who have a less aggressive viral form.

The **vaccines against HPV** available today represent a safe and effective prevention tool. The quadrivalent vaccine (against HPV 6, 11, 16 and 18) introduced in Italy in 2008 has reduced infections by 89% among girls between fourteen and twenty-four, as well as partially develop what we've come to know as herd immunity, in which those without vaccines are potentially protected. There's also the 9-valent vaccine, which has an even broader range of action and is now recommended.

We often hear talk about female vaccination, but it's important for males to get vaccinated as well. Every Italian region acts differently on this front. On the website www.ioscelgo.it you'll find precise information concerning the vaccine's cost (if any) and the clinics that offer it.

Unlike women, who need to get vaccinated prior to their first sexual experience, men can get vaccinated at any age. In 2007 I coauthored a study on male vaccination against HPV which won the award for Best European Urological Scientific Paper and which medical science is still discussing to this day.

As I think we've clarified, screening is important for preventing the spread of sexually-transmitted diseases. And the pap-test for women and HPV DNA test are the only two methods available to us. As for the other tumors associated with HPV infection, at the moment there are no ad hoc screening programs, but vaccination remains a valid prevention tool for everyone. Acts of good sense, like getting vaccinated and correctly using condoms, allow you to avoid potentially serious complications. Vaccination against HPV doesn't protect against other sexually-transmitted diseases: the recommendation to always use condoms is valid for those who've been vaccinated too.

Genital Herpes

When we talk about herpes we immediately think of the lips. Genital herpes, even if visually similar to the labial variety, differs in the type of virus that causes the infection. The genital disease is induced by an infection of type-2 Herpes Simplex Virus (HSV-2), while the labial sort comes from HSV-I.

One of the first warning signs of genital herpes is the appearance of small red or white vesicles on the glans, the foreskin and even the skin of the shaft, and in women in the vulvar mucous. In more virulent cases, the pustules can extend to the thighs and perianal area. There may also be fever.

Generally, the lesions evolve into rather painful micro-ulcers, often covered by little scabs, as occurs on the lips as well. Infection, as in Gabriel's case (the protagonist of the story on p. 118), takes place because some carriers of the virus don't develop visible symptoms and aren't aware they're contagious.

Treatment can be localized through the use of anti-herpes creams, or oral medications that fight the infection from within. The positive thing is that—as with labial herpes—the visible lesions heal in a few days, at most a few weeks, without leaving a trace, though the affected area may remain sensitive to the touch for a prolonged period.

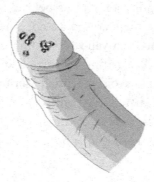

Figure n. 17—Appearance of Genital Herpes

Hepatitis B and C

Lastly, there are the **Hepatitis B and Hepatitis C** viruses, transmittable through exchanges of blood.

They are difficult to contract during intercourse, since infection occurs more frequently in situations in which blood is directly involved.

But the possibility cannot be entirely excluded, and the forms of protection used against other STDs function against these forms of hepatitis as well, even if we're not aware of it.

The First Time Is Forever

I rush into my office after a morning in the operating room. As usual, I consult the list of patients and the last name sounds familiar.

When it's his turn, I open the door and come face to face with my friend Maurizio and his sixteen-year-old son Gabriele, whom I've known since he was little. Gabriele, who immediately looks very worried, insists on speaking to me alone, so I wave him in, gesturing at his father to wait outside. At this point I ask him bluntly what the problem is.

He tells me, very serious and determined: "Well, I had sex for the first time last week."

I imagine that he's looking for advice and that his father, embarrassed, delegated the task to me. But he surprises me. He tells me that two days ago he noticed some painful blisters appear on his glans.

The first question I ask him is obligatory: "Did you use a condom?"

Timidly he answers no, because his girlfriend Greta, the same age as him, whom he's been seeing for a month, told him that she'd only had one previous experience and plus he doesn't know how to use one. I examine him and the diagnosis is clear: genital herpes.

At this point I bring Maurizio in to tell them both the situation. The treatment calls for oral antivirals and the local application of an ointment. Unfortunately, even after the disappearance of the symptoms, the virus remains latent in the organism for the rest of your life, so the person who has it can both infect their partner and be subject to relapses, particularly when immune defenses are low, thus making it necessary to begin the treatment all over again. A boy this young will have serious repercussions in the future, which might not place him in danger but will influence his quality of life.

Gabriele is pretty angry and asks me how it's possible that his girlfriend doesn't have symptoms, insisting on the fact that she'd only had one prior sexual experience. The answer I give him is that the virus attacks our organism subjectively and even if his girlfriend doesn't have any visible symptoms she ought to see a gynecologist for treatment. In this regard, in my talks at schools, I often repeat a concept that I deem very important: if your partner has had intercourse a hundred times but always used a condom, they're safer than someone who has had it only once without protection. Condoms are synonymous with respect for yourself and your partner.

BACTERIAL SEXUALLY-TRANSMITTED DISEASES

Syphilis

With a long and pervasive history, syphilis was widespread in the West from the Renaissance until the last century. It is often mentioned in literature and art, and its victims include author Guy de Maupassant and artist Paul Gauguin.

Caused by the bacterium *Treponema pallidum*, according to one of the most authoritative hypotheses it may have reached Europe with the sailors who accompanied Christopher Columbus on the discovery of the New World. What's certain is that it still affects millions of people today—twelve million at the beginning of the century, mainly in developing countries—particularly between the ages of fifteen and twenty, and that it's one of the main causes of miscarriages.

The first symptom in men is a small **ulcer on the penis.** Ulcers are sores that can form on the glans or the inside of the foreskin. They indicate the existence of an underlying pathology, even a simple infection, in correspondence with which there will be a serous secretion containing bacteria. There are different types, each indicating a different pathology.

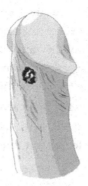

Figure n. 18—Syphilis Sores

If they're precursors of syphilis, they appear isolated. In that case, the ulcer is round or oval, and not particularly painful. They can, however, be connected to other rarer diseases, such as **venereal lymphogranuloma,** a sexually-transmitted infection caused by the chlamydia bacterium. In addition to the ulcer, in this case we note a swelling of the inguinal lymph nodes, which in turn often form dermatological lesions. Finally, **tumoral ulcers** appear with hard and irregular edges and are very painful.

If treated immediately, the disease isn't difficult to overcome. The ulcer can heal on its own, but this doesn't mean that the disease is cured, since it can persist in a latent form. To resolve it, an antibiotics-based therapy for several days will suffice. If neglected, on the other hand, it can become extremely dangerous, and in a range between 8% and 58% of cases can even lead to death.

Gonorrhea

Once known as "the clap," and in Italian as *scolo* ("drain") from the most visible symptom, the loss of urine and pus, gonorrhea can affect the genitals of both men and women. Precarious hygienic conditions, dietary insufficiencies, lack of medical assistance, sexual promiscuity and failure to use condoms are among the principal causes. At its most aggressive, it can even attack other parts of the body, from the rectum to the pharynx, the joints, the liver, even the myocardium.

This, too, can be treated with antibiotics, to be started as soon as possible partly to prevent the triggering of a concurrent syphilis infection.

Chlamydia, Ureaplasma and Mycoplasma

Here we group three bacterial infections that appear with the same symptom: **itching and irritation during urination,** and **urethritis,** an acute or chronic inflammation of the urethra.

The diagnosis is made via a urethral swab.

Infection from *chlamydia trachomatis* is the most sexually frequent in Europe. But all three of them are treatable with specific antibiotics, prescribed by a urologist or family doctor.

Yeast Infection

Completing the picture, finally, is the yeast infection from *candida albicans*, a fungus present in our organism whose aggression is generally triggered by an alteration in the immune defenses. It can be transmitted by sexual partners, but usually isn't classified as a sexually-transmitted disease. Even if it's more frequent in women, in men it can cause irritation and burning under the foreskin, **balanitis** (inflammation of the glans), or the appearance of red splotches or tiny sores.

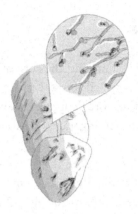

Figure n. 19—*Candida albicans* Sores

The heavy use of antibiotics to fight any normal sort of infection can create the appropriate conditions for the fungus to proliferate, thus setting off a vicious cycle: the treatment of one problem generates another problem, and so on. I recommend the use of specific genital cleansers and anti-fungal creams.

Many of these pathologies have similar symptoms and can be difficult to recognize. This makes it even more important to see an expert, capable of accurately identifying the virus, bacterium or fungus and prescribing the most appropriate treatment.

This treatment must then be extended to the partner(s) with whom the person has had intercourse. Informing the people with whom we've had sex so that they can be tested and treated is the responsible thing to do.

Let me also repeat that prevention can be done in two ways: getting vaccinated and, as you now know by heart, using a condom.

EMERGENCIES

Emergencies are just around the corner in adolescence as well. Experimenting, as we all know, can lead to disastrous results. Reader beware: the word "rupture" is about to appear multiple times. For all these emergencies, go to the nearest ER as soon as possible.

The **rupture of the frenulum** occurs when the band of skin is too short (frenulum breve) and the condition was not identified and resolved medically. The accident can occur all of a sudden, rarely during masturbation and more often during the first sexual experiences. The rupture is followed by bleeding, sometimes copious. You can react by staunching the area in question and thus blocking the small hemorrhage. If you're unable to, you'll require stitches. In either case, seeing a specialist is recommended.

The **fracture of the penis**, sometimes playfully referred to as "broken nail syndrome," is a more serious trauma. What breaks is the tunica albuginea that protects the corpora cavernosa, generally during the sexual act, since the penis has to be erect.

What a Ball-Breaker

It's four o'clock on a summer afternoon and at the clinic there's an almost surreal calm, I've gotten one cancellation after another. Just as I start thinking about what to eat for dinner, the letters "ECD" appear on my cellphone screen: Emergency and Check-In Department. In other words: ER.

"What is it?"

"Hurry, we have a boy with a serious trauma, the testicle is one big bruise, I've never seen anything like it." Rushing down the stairs, I alert the operating room and ask the anesthesiologist to be sent to the ER. When I get there, I realize why the nurse was so agitated on the phone. The boy's right testicle is dark blue.

Niccolò is seventeen, a motocross champion, and he's had an accident in a race. His dad Massimiliano is desperate. I inform him that we'll have to operate on the fractured testicle and evaluate the seriousness of the damage.

The young man stares at me, white as a sheet; his father Massimiliano won't accept it.

"He just banged it! It was practically nothing, do you know how many times my friends hit me in the balls and I was in awful pain for a few minutes and then I was fine? Shouldn't we just put some ice on it? Aren't there alternatives to operating?"

"No, there aren't, trust me, and let's avoid making this experience any more complex than it already is. I need your and your wife's authorization immediately, seeing as Niccolò is a minor."

After an hour of phone calls and arguments we're in the operating room. Enrico, my colleague and friend, has arrived as well. We try to drain the hematic effusion, but the scrotal structure is seriously compromised. The testicle can't be saved, we have to remove it.

I see the boy a month later, at the post-op check-up, accompanied by his mom who apologizes to me for her husband's behavior after the operation. Massimiliano had refused to speak with me, in fact it looked like he was suffering more than Niccolò. We schedule a smaller, second operation that morning to position a prosthetic testicle. He asks me lots of questions and I reassure him: no one will notice the presence of a fake silicone testicle, and his fertility will be normal even with just one, after all, that's why nature gave us two! Together we decide on the correct size of the prosthesis and it's all over in just over than twenty minutes.

A few months later I get an email with an attached photo of Niccolò soaring through the air on his motorbike. A red circle highlights his race number: 2. Only after do I read the body of the message.

Luckily there's two of them! Thanks, doc! Niccolò.

I smile and forward the photo to Enrico, sharing the happy ending to this terrible experience.

Studies have found that it's much more frequent when intercourse takes place in stressful conditions or in an uncomfortable place that forces you to put yourself in awkward positions for the sexual act, such as in a car. You become aware of it principally due to the sharp pain, but a crunching sound can also be heard, as though it were a bone. The rupture of the tunica causes an effusion of blood, which is why you see bruises or darker zones.

The only solution in this case is surgery. Under general anesthesia, an incision is made in the penis to repair the lesion, followed by roughly ten stitches. After this operation it's necessary to abstain from sexual intercourse until healing is complete.

When I hear the expression "What a ballbreaker!" I don't always think of the figurative sense of the expression. Various testicular traumas are possible, in fact, including **rupture**, as we saw in Niccolò's case, which is different than **torsion**, which we discussed vis-à-vis childhood. Blows to the testicles generate some of the most intense pain a man can feel. Sometimes the impact wears off after a few minutes, or by applying ice, other times it can persist at length. In the latter cases it's best to see a doctor, because only an ultrasound can confirm the rupture of the testicle.

Contact sports and being hit with a ball are among the most common causes, such that an added layer of protection is often recommended: reinforced underwear or a jock strap, as in boxing.

Then there are **burns**. We've already mentioned the improper use of depilatory wax, which remains one of the most frequent causes of genital burns, but the most ordinary accidents are just around the corner. In the ER, I treated patients who burned themselves with boiling pasta water or an iron on numerous occasions. Nor should plain old bad luck be underestimated in these cases.

Doctors' responsibility is to be available to our patients, their problems, their questions and their concerns, well-founded or otherwise. It isn't rare, in fact, for some latent pathology to be caught early during a routine check-up or emergency admission. Common sense, paying attention, prevention, and openness to dialogue and exchange are key factors for resolving most problems discussed here, and are essential for any process of identifying and resolving health issues for adolescents, but they are extremely useful in the relationship with adults as well.

3

THE ADULT PENIS

"This cock of mine's a tiger! It's ferocious, it's powerful! What help could it possibly need?" writes a thirty-nine-year-old dad in response to a survey on the frequency of male reproductive system checkups. Then he corrects himself: "Oh, what an awful thing to write."

"Adulthood: the period in a person's life that begins at the end of adolescence and continues until the start of old age. It's composed of a first phase that corresponds with youth (20–30) and maturity (30–45) and a second stage, that of middle age (45–65)."

This is PerFormat Salute's definition of an adult.

I immediately feel like saying: what a long stage! From the end of adolescence, the adult male body remains nearly the same for roughly thirty years, undergoing small alterations or modifications that generally occur over the age of fifty. In this long period the penis remains unchanged as well, in a condition of stability, before the onset of old age.

So this is going to be a dense chapter. It includes many crucial phases of sexuality, fertility, and our relationship with medication.

Our division into Upkeep, Pathologies and Emergencies remains,
but we'll also dedicate significant space to the Covid-19 pandemic
and its repercussions.

Forever Young

"I saw a photo of you dressed as Batman on the internet!"

It's Antonio, scheduled for an operation with me tomorrow. I thought he was calling with routine pre-surgery questions. I stammer: "I really apologize . . . I'll ask a colleague to replace me."

"No, no, don't do that! I'm thrilled that Batman's operating on me! And while I have you here, how long did you say it's going to take?"

Now I want to explain the existence of this photo.

A few years ago a dear friend of mine asked me to help him on a project for a photography contest entitled "The Fall of the Superheroes."

"Listen, would you happen to have two other friends as crazy as you who are willing to spend Saturday afternoon in costume? I want to photograph three superheroes who've fallen on hard times."

"Sure, no problem." When a friend asks for help, you do what you can.

Three days later Franco, Gerardo and I became Batman, Superman and Spiderman. In the flesh.

"Gerry, we're in downtown Florence, what do I do if I run into someone I know?"

Before I can even finish the sentence I hear a voice. "Hey, Doc! Why are you in costume today?

It's April, Carnival's been over for a while now!" It's a patient, and he's speaking to me from the driver's seat of his car.

"Yes, look . . . would you please stop honking and drive, we're blocking traffic. And don't forget your therapy, you've got a check-up in a month."

We're pulling away from the "De Amicis" stop on the n. 6 bus line when a woman of around seventy sits down next to us and, without batting an eye, asks for information on the bus schedule.

Maybe I should wear that costume more often. I feel as if it corresponds to the image of the adult I'd like to be, free from constrictions.

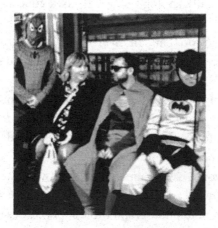

UPKEEP

The social importance of **penile hygiene** abruptly diminishes as boys become men. Advertising doesn't help: on TV there are only ads for female genital itching, cleansing with pink bottles and women's urinary leakage, while Adonis-like bodies take center stage in razor and aftershave ads. I don't think I'm unveiling any secrets if I say that in the public opinion there are still double standards for women and men when it comes to genital hygiene, care, routines and rituals. In truth it really shouldn't be up for debate: a clean penis is a healthier penis, and the same goes for a vagina. Noticing strange smells despite correct hygiene can be a sign of the fact that something's wrong. An infection or a modification of the glans's bacterial flora might be underway. Phimosis can be another cause of an unpleasant odor, causing difficulties in cleansing and an accumulation of urine or smegma. Remember to wash! Always taking care not to use soaps that are too strong (no, three-in-one soap-shampoo-deodorants are not recommended). Today we can clone our penis to turn it into a sex toy, wear padded underwear to fool the curious into thinking we have an extra-large schlong, but there's no place except the urologist's clinic where we can feel free to talk about the subject frankly. This book aims to bring a bit of the atmosphere of my office into the houses of you readers (but onto the beach as well, it depends on where you read it). It's crucial to set off a virtuous cycle, so that little by little we abandon the idea that the health of the penis and everything that revolves around it is taboo, particularly among the people concerned.

During adulthood the penis doesn't undergo any substantial morphological changes, except if pathologies set in. Last chapter's recommendation to conduct a self-examination of the testicles once a month remains as valid as ever, though this practice certainly isn't widespread in Italy due to the lack of information. Testicular cancer, in fact, strikes most aggressively in the age range from twenty to forty, while it's rarer after sixty: without a self-examination and looking at yourself in the mirror it's almost impossible to diagnose the tumor at an early stage.

Here's a **brief guide on how to conduct a testicular checkup**. It only takes a few minutes. Delicately slide each testicle between your thumb and index finger. Touch its entire surface. Its consistency should all be uniform (remember that it's normal for one testicle to be slightly larger than the other).

Let's play doctor and look for the epididymis and the vasa deferentia: they are soft structures, similar to small tubes, above and behind the testicle, and they serve to transport the spermatozoa. Familiarize yourself with the feeling of these cords. Look for clots, swellings, something that seems out of place, even if it doesn't cause pain.

The check-up needs to be conducted at least once a month. We need to pay attention to any change in size, shape or consistency, and if we notice a nodule or anything else, see a doctor. Maybe it's nothing, but if it turns out to be a tumor it could spread very quickly, and if the diagnosis is made in time we can get treatment, at least in 99% of cases.

Who knows how many articles entitled "Love in the Time of the Coronavirus" you've run into lately. I've read lots of them. So much has been said about the coronavirus itself and its means of transmission, the vaccine and everything connected to them. But here, in my own little garden, I'd like to dedicate a few more words to the implications that Covid has had and will have in the urological and sexual realms.

My first interview in this regard dates back to March 5, 2020, two weeks after the discovery of the first case in Italy, on Radio24's show "La Zanzara." The message I wanted to get out was that, sure, making love raised immune defenses, but in that specific phase it was necessary to choose one single partner, or, worst-case scenario, go solo. The question was completely ignored. During the first lockdown TV was besieged by a whole series of virologists and immunologists who left our emotional sphere in the background for a simple reason: Covid doesn't have direct repercussions on sexuality.

The question, as always, is a little more complex. Studies and research conducted from the beginning of the pandemic have highlighted something that is worth taking into consideration and whose fallout we'll note later on: the **implications of Covid in the field of urology** are distinguishable mainly in the area of sexuality and in that of tumoral pathologies.

The data reveal that in the first lockdown in the couples interviewed in the study "The Impact of the Covid-19 Quarantine on Sexual Life in Italy" there was an increase in sexual desire of 40%, as the same was true for auto-eroticism. On the contrary, there was a fall in sexual satisfaction (-53%). Even the frequency of monthly sexual relations followed the same trend, despite the greater amount of time available with one's partner. People also didn't experiment much in bed, preferring to trust in habit, a lifeboat amid the tsunami.

The sexologists who looked into this paradox found a reasonable explanation in what in jargon is defined as "parentalization": spending time together while *completely* forgetting about seduction. This causes great difficulty in seeing the other person as a lover, but more as a sister or brother. A high percentage of interviewees also says they became closer to their partner and argued with them less. This is natural if we consider the fact that we had to grapple with the fear of losing someone that we loved and with the need to preserve domestic tranquility that we were forced to share. But there weren't the necessary conditions for this particularly intense affection to lead to sex.

The couple most in crisis were undoubtedly those in which both partners were used to spending the day outside of the home for work. Being forced to spend the whole day together upset the dynamics of the couple; in addition to the trouble in facing one's own personal crises it was also necessary to make room for the other person's. In short, nothing new in the relationship field; what changed was the intensity.

The couple who had or will have the strength to ask for help from psychologists, sexologists and therapists are already halfway there. Love isn't always enough, particularly in an absurd situation like the one in which we found ourselves from one day to the next.

Then there are those who experienced a long-distance relationship, who say they made recourse to long sessions of sexting and Zoom calls in the attempt to keep the little flame of excitement alive. Sex-toy producers even used their ingenuity to create devices that could be remotely controlled . . . now that's "adaptability."

We witnessed an increase in the use of pornography, verifiable as well from the search data of Google users. Among other things, as you'll remember, Pornhub decided to sacrifice itself for the cause and give away free premium subscriptions to Italians, making the hashtag #iorestoacasa ("I'm staying home") a little spicier. Sales of drugs against erectile dysfunction fell, on the other hand, bearing witness to the fact that opportunities to use them, due in part to the distance of our partners, maybe in another town, had been drastically reduced.

At the end of the first quarantine, when optimism and the hashtag #andràtuttobene ("Everything will be fine") was just a distant memory, there was an increase in states of depression and anxiety, which naturally had even more negative repercussions on the sexual sphere. So if before people were already not making love much and with little satisfaction, in the second lockdown the situation grew even darker. Just as Google searches about impotence and erectile dysfunction diminished, so did those about fertility and the desire to be parents. Thinking about expanding our family in uncertain times was not in fact a priority, at least for most Italians. Recourse to artificial insemination also fell, due to the need to avoid the overcrowded hospitals. As far as pathologies are concerned, on the other hand, in the coming years we will see a growth in the number of tumors, including that of the prostate. The reason is to be sought in the fall, in truth the near-total absence, of all those preventive checkups and screenings that were postponed as "not urgent" and which are actually crucial for discovering them in time, before they degenerate. My advice: as soon as you can, reschedule all the appointments that you avoided making to keep away from the hospitals.

Remaining in the area of specific prevention, we've decided to insert in the section dedicated to upkeep the analyses that concern **prostate cancer**, to underline the importance of the diagnosis and check-ups rather than its development as a pathology.

Prostate cancer is one of the most common forms of cancer in the male population: the probability of developing it is equal to one in eight. But this needn't be a cause for alarm. Recovery rates are promising, particularly when you intervene quickly: 90% of patients treated are still alive five years after the diagnosis, which is a positive datum.

I want to repeat yet again that prevention and early diagnosis are fundamental. In this case genetics takes on an important role: the risk of prostate cancer doubles if a close relative has had an analogous tumor (a father or brother, but also a mother or sister with breast or ovarian cancer, for which the same genetic mutations are responsible) and it's precisely for this reason that it's fundamental to be watchful and monitor yourself. Even **lifestyle** can influence the possibilities of developing a tumor: for example a diet rich in saturated fats and sedentary behavior can favor it. Lastly, **aging** is another factor. Before forty we're still in an age range in which it's premature to worry if there are no symptoms, but after forty-five it's necessary.

Among the warning signs of prostate cancer, which is asymptomatic in the early stages, are problems during urination, including pain and burning. Blood in the urine or sperm, the need to urinate frequently at night and difficulties in maintaining a constant flow ought to push us to ask questions and take a closer look. All these symptoms, as we'll see later, can also be associated with other, potentially benign prostate pathologies.

The tumor's diagnosis takes place via a rectal exam, to be conducted in a urologist or family doctor's office, but the PSA test is also a good indicator. In fact the prostate is the only gland characterized by a personalized marker—the PSA, or Prostate-Specific Antigen—that alerts you to whether some pathology has arisen in its gland. More concretely, the PSA is the enzyme produced by the prostate which serves to keep sperm fluid after ejaculation.

Analysis of the PSA occurs through a blood test that doesn't require fasting, but in the forty-eight hours beforehand it's best to abstain from intense physical activity because this could distort the results. It's always good to remember that an abnormal level doesn't automatically imply a tumor. According to the data, indeed, in 75% of cases with elevated PSA the subsequent biopsy doesn't reveal a tumor, but rather an anomaly. The main aspect of the exam is given by the indicator's variation over time. This is why it's important to take a first PSA test around 45–50 and then repeat it at regular intervals so as to monitor its changes. Today it's even possible to take it at the pharmacy through a capillary blood test: you get your result in fifteen minutes.

Taking the exam constantly over one's life makes it possible to understand the marker's evolution in the individual. If, for example, we see a sudden and significant rise, we're probably in the presence of a transitory inflammation, rather than a tumor. A slow and constant increase could indicate a benign prostatic hyperplasia. Going from 2.5 to 2.9, on the other hand, should suggest the wisdom of taking a closer look: even if it might appear to be in the norm, this modification could indicate that a tumoral cell has formed or is forming.

Once you've measured your PSA, you need to see a urologist who will "read" the data. Only he can interpret the shifts: avoid doing so yourself. The PSA isn't the gas meter, the question is far more complex. The data gathered must be combined with the patient's clinical profile, personal history, family history, and the exam at the clinic.

With monitoring and good prevention, all situations can be resolved in a positive manner. The next time you see your family doctor, have them prescribe this test for you.

A bit ago we were mentioning the desire to become parents, an argument that's intimately linked to that of **fertility**. Wanting to leave a tangible mark on our planet is stressful for many of us, and one of the solutions for satisfying it is having children, thus contributing to the continuation of the species: roughly 85% of couples who try to conceive, engaging regularly in sexual relations without using contraception, obtain a pregnancy within a year. But the remaining 15 percent encounter problems.

Increasing Intimacy

Antonio is forty years old, Silvia thirty-five, they've been together for five years and have decided that it's time to bring their first child into the world. He's an architect and lives in Milan, while she, a lawyer, lives in Florence. Even after getting married they've maintained their long-distance relationship: they're happy about what they've managed to build, both as a couple—they're very proud of the intensity of their relationship—and personally, because their independence has led them to two brilliant careers.

They come to my clinic after a frustrating year trying to get pregnant, convinced that something in one of them isn't working. They've come to me to find out whether the problem is Antonio's or Silvia's.

They tell me their story, but I stop them as they tell me about their separate residences.

"How often do you see each other?" I ask.

"On Skype almost every night, to keep each other company while we eat; in person on Saturday and Sunday, sometimes here in Florence and other times at my place, we take turns."

"Well, there's your problem."

Their faces look extremely perplexed. Antonio falls silent and crosses his arms, Silvia stares me down and raises her voice. "Hey, listen, we're here for a medical consultation. I already have to put up with the sermons of my mother, who says that we can't keep this up, that a married woman shouldn't live alone, that Antonio's cheating on me. I have no intention of getting the sermon from you as well. The choice is ours alone, we'll be the ones to decide what's right for us, got it?"

"Hold on, if you let me explain I'm sure we can clear up this misunderstanding. I have absolutely no intention of taking your mother's place," I reply. "When aspiring parents come to see me, exhausted by a pregnancy that won't come, I always use a comparison that I think is very effective: having a child is like shooting at a target, sometimes it's just luck, sometimes you need to practice. Increasing your attempts increases your chances of success. After all, getting pregnant is a statistical matter. Your target shooting, due to the physical distance that separates you, is comparable more to a hobby than a serious sport. I don't want to judge, but just tell you that from a medical standpoint your attempts are too few to reach the conclusion that something isn't working."

The situation has calmed down a bit. I tell them that we'll proceed with all the appropriate clinical evaluations, first a sperm test for Antonio and then a gynecological visit for Silvia.

A month later, with the test results that everything is functioning properly, I insist once more on the need to spend more time together to have more intercourse. In my office a new debate begins, but different than the last one.

"Listen, Silvia, come live with me, there's no way I can leave work, we have too many ongoing projects and Lorenzo wouldn't understand . . ."

"I already told you that I can't just leave, with all the sacrifices I've made I can't just take off now."

"Silvia, come on, you know perfectly well that . . ."

I'm saved by a knock at the door from the clinic's assistant. "Doctor, Mr. Cecchinelli called, he wants to know if he can move up his five o'clock."

The two of them stand up without another word and walk out, visibly agitated. The confirmation that their numbers are all in the norm may have been a more bitter pill to swallow than some problem with a medical solution.

In June I see Antonio again after several months, this time for a pain in a testicle that turns out to be nothing more than a blow he received in a friendly basketball game, it'll pass on its own in a few days. I take the opportunity to ask about the situation with Silvia. Antonio tells me that nothing has changed.

"If I may, it could be useful to take advantage of your summer vacation that's around the corner to spend at least three weeks together, without anyone around." Antonio doesn't look very persuaded by the suggestion, and I get the sense that I won't see or hear from him again.

In September I get a text with an attachment, a selfie in the Tuscan hills.

It worked!

If, unlike Antonio and Silvia, you've conscientiously tried time and again to no avail, it could be useful to consider investigating the causes and, subsequently, the appropriate treatment. In delicate moments like this, full of dread, it's necessary for both partners to speak frankly of their expectations and willingness to undertake a specific process.

Today there are very sophisticated technologies to treat most causes of infertility. But the success rates for some of these are nowhere near 100 percent. Some couples choose to remain childless and this is an understandable choice. But it's important that any decision be mutual. If you intend to proceed with treatment, have some idea of how far you want to go with it. Infertility treatments can be expensive, long, painful, and in some cases can fail. It's useful to establish your limit right from the beginning.

Any investigation into fertility should consider the couple as a unit. Personally I believe that the root of the problem of having trouble getting pregnant should first be sought in the man, for the simple fact that it's faster to assemble a clinical picture of the situation. Examination, hormone tests, ultrasound, cultural tests and spermiogram are quick, exhaustive and dependable steps. In roughly 30 percent of cases of infertility the cause is solely male and in another 20 percent the problem lies with both parties.

The man is thus involved in 50 percent of cases. Though we should specify: analyzing the problems of females will not be dealt with here simply because they lie outside of my realm of expertise.

The first thing to be done is a spermiogram in a specialized lab. We're asked to ejaculate into a container, behind closed doors (once upon a time pornographic magazines were provided, but now we rely on the internet), just before the analysis of the sperm sample—no more than two hours before—because it's important to verify the mobility of the spermatozoa, more than their quantity (how well they can swim and thus find their path through the uterus and into the Fallopian tube, in a sort of Cooper test). The recommendation is to abstain from sex for a period of two to five days beforehand—I always personally suggest two or three, in order to obtain a "rich" sample.

A low number of spermatozoa, a reduced mobility or other anomalies will require the test to be repeated, possibly more than once. If we detect a persistent anomaly it doesn't mean that we cannot inseminate: the diagnosis of infertility occurs only if the absence of spermatozoa (**azoospermia**) is constant.

The causes of a certain difficulty in fertilizing can be diverse, but among the most recurrent are the use of certain medicines, steroids or other hormones, drug and alcohol abuse, exposure to radiation, chromosomal anomalies, hormonal problems, a pre-existing parotitis, a hemochromatosis, or the progressive accumulation of iron in the organism (roughly 80 percent of men with this pathology report testicular malfunctioning), a pre-existing testicular or penile trauma, incompletely-descended testicles and **varicocele**.

Varicocele is the most frequent cause, because the increased testicular temperature and the interference with the blood flow by the varicose veins prevents a good production of spermatozoa. This is generally resolved through surgery, very similar to that varicose veins in the legs. It doesn't guarantee a total resolution of the problem, but together with monitoring the number of spermatozoa and their mobility through lab tests it can be a step forward.

One of the most frequent chromosomal anomalies in sperm is **Klinefelter's syndrome**, affecting one out of seven hundred men. Infertility in these individuals is due to the development of fibrous tissue and the thickening of the testicles and can be treatable if discovered at a young age, yet is only diagnosed in one-fourth of cases.

The most common warning signs appear during puberty, when the development of the penis is complete but the testicles remain relatively small. We can also notice it if we observe a tall stature, longer-than-normal upper limbs and, in some individuals, a gynecomastia, or an increase in mammary fat; also, the lack of facial hair and the tendency to accumulate fat in the lower part of the body such as gynoid males (in short, the tendency to take on a "pear-shaped" appearance).

There is no resolutory treatment for the syndrome, but you can make recourse to testosterone injections to help the secondary sexual characteristics develop. As far as evaluating fertility is concerned, it's necessary as usual to go to a specialized center. Certain individuals require a sperm sample and the cryo-preservation of the testicle's pubescent spermatogonia, to make possible in the future, should you desire, to proceed to in-vitro fertilization, though the results aren't guaranteed.

As for external factors, on the other hand, on the one hand the improved medical and hygienic conditions in which we live have eliminated a long list of pathologies and risk factors for the reproductive system as well; on the other, we're immersed in an environment that bombards us with substances and endangers the vitality of our spermatozoa. The air we breathe, particularly in cities, is an almost trite example, but what we eat counts a great deal as well. If DDT and chemical additives have undergone an apparent regression in recent years, we continue to find on our plates pesticides and microplastics to a worrying extent. Unfortunately phthalates—the chemical compounds of plastics in packaging—along with pesticides and estrogen, negatively influence a man's hormonal balance, stimulating strong anti-androgenic consequences.

But that's not all. Urology, too, is influenced by climate change. It's now proven that an increase of one degree in the environmental temperature raises scrotal temperature by 0.1 degrees. Such a variation can compromise male fertility . . . planet Earth isn't the only "ball" being overheated. Difficulties getting pregnant depend not only on clinical or psychological reasons, but also on environmental and nutritional factors. This is confirmed by a study that has compared spermiograms of twenty years ago with those of today: overall, the number of spermatozoa appears to have diminished.

Should these continue to be low in number or simply not sufficiently active, and after doing all the proper genetic, behavioral and pathological analyses, our semen can be assisted by technologies such as **artificial insemination, in vitro fertilization** (IVF) or **Intracytoplasmic Sperm Injection** (ICSI). ICSI consists of obtaining a sperm sample through ejaculation into a container or aspiration from within the testicle with a needle, after the administration of an anesthetic. This is undertaken when there are problems of obstruction in the complex hydraulic system that brings the spermatozoa from the testicles to the penis. The sample is then injected directly into the egg taken from the woman's body, which, fertilized, is implanted in her uterus.

The procedure's success rate is around 30 percent.

Artificial insemination with sperm donated from a sperm bank is also a possibility. In Italy there are few of them and accessible only to heterosexual couples. If you choose to proceed in this direction a meticulous consultation and a thorough discussion with your partner, since the child conceived will have a different biological father, even if unknown. It will then be the child's right to know their genetic history.

With both IVF and ICSI it's necessary to accept that a successful implantation of the embryo doesn't ensure a successful pregnancy. As in natural pregnancies, in these, too, there can be miscarriages, and it's thus necessary to keep in mind the psychological implications of this unfruitful effort. Many couples, after the first miscarriage, decide not to attempt a second time and choose adoption or foster parenting, equally valid paths which, however, present their own array of obstacles.

SEXUALLY-TRANSMITTED PATHOLOGIES

In adulthood as well, we need to focus our attention on **sexually-transmitted diseases.** We discussed them in the chapter on adolescence, but we do so again here because they also appear with great frequency among adults, particularly due to misinformation. A teenager who doesn't use condoms properly will be a neglectful adult. In fact, the phenomenon of "sexual nomadism" is perhaps even more intense in this period, so recommendations on the importance of using condoms are obligatory.

Lesser attention to precautions—evident after the great fear caused by AIDS at the end of the last century—might be reversed in the current situation and in the post-COVID era. We've grown used to the idea that gloves and masks are useful against viruses, and so using condoms might come more naturally too. It would be a positive development given that, due to the intense migratory influxes from Africa and South America, a whole series of pathologies that until a short time ago seemed to have been uprooted in Europe are reappearing—**syphilis, gonococcal infection, chlamydia, gonorrhea**. They often appear as **urethritis,** or a burning sensation during urination, accompanied in some cases by the emergence of a pus-like material from the penis: in such cases, see a specialist immediately. Therapy calls for treating the cause via antibiotics, antivirals or antifungals, depending on the type of infection.

Fortunately, in recent years there has been a profound evolution in diagnostic techniques, such that today we can recognize what used to pass for a simple inflammation. But cases of STDs in this age range are still quite numerous.

NON-SEXUALLY-TRANSMITTED PATHOLOGIES

Phimosis

We mention **phimosis**—already discussed for children and adolescents—since it can actually appear during any stage of life, and in adults assumes a peculiar profile. When foreskin shrinkage suddenly appears in an adult male, there are only three possible causes: diabetes, lichen sclerosus, balanitis.

A patient who has suffered from **diabetes** from birth or has developed the nutritional form—Type-2 Diabetes—may in time develop phimosis. The closed penis, in this case, is merely a sign of a more general situation that must be resolved via tests and ad hoc therapies.

In the adult male **lichen sclerosus** is simple to recognize, since the foreskin takes on specific colors and morphologies, with a dominance of whitish parts. This is a non-contagious dermatological condition whose origin isn't perfectly clear. The most recent theories point to hereditary factors, hormonal imbalances or immune system dysfunctions.

The spots covering the affected area are initially glossy and flat, then tend to dry up and rupture, leaving bruising and scarring. Their appearance is associated with other symptoms, including itching in the affected areas, pain, blisters or bleeding. Since the cause is unknown, treatment is based on cortisone creams. More serious cases can require the lesion's surgical removal.

This penile closure, finally, can also occur due to untreated infections, mainly bacterial or mycotic (**balanitis**). In this case there's only a localized solution: surgical circumcision.

Erectile Dysfunction

Also appearing in this phase are **erectile dysfunction** and **premature ejaculation**, by far the most talked-about subjects in my professional life.

Let's start by debunking the myth that the penis stops functioning all of a sudden. **Erectile dysfunction** deserves a more thorough discussion. First of all, it's a symptom, and if it only appears occasionally it's no cause for alarm.

When I explain it to my students, I begin by comparing it with coughing.

Coughing is a symptom. If it only happens once, in the morning, it might not mean anything; if it lasts for several days, it's best to see your family doctor to make sure it isn't bronchitis. If it persists after a mild therapy, further radiological tests are carried out which can lead to serious diagnoses such as pneumonia or, in extreme cases, lung or pleural cancer.

The same is true for erectile dysfunction: if the symptom persists, a medical specialist should intervene to achieve a clear diagnosis.

It's a good idea to run further tests in part because they can lead to diagnoses that go beyond sexuality to other aspects of our life.

The erectile mechanism is synonymous with overall health, so the systematic presence of this sort of problem shouldn't be underestimated. Sexual activity, in fact, is an important component of an individual's well-being, regardless of gender: even if sporadic, it permits the release of endorphins and a whole series of other mediators that relax the mind and the entire organism, benefitting even the immune system.

Men struggle to talk about conditions that regard their intimate sphere, whether these are emotional or physical. This is true even in their own mind: they prefer to explain things away as fatigue or an off-night. And believe me, it's no different at the specialist's office. It takes them an average of three years to reach full awareness.

Firstly, it's good to be clear about what erectile dysfunction means scientifically.

As we've seen, the penis's normal erections are caused by a variety of stimuli. The mechanism is the same, no matter what excites us. Our brain, acting through the involuntary nervous system, triggers an alteration in the flow of blood to the penis. The tissue of the corpora cavernosa relax and allow the blood to fill them, causing the penis to enlarge, straighten and raise up.

The classic simile is a sponge filling up with water. Until this magic circuit is interrupted or reaches its climax with ejaculation, the penis remains erect.

But many things can interfere. A lesser ability to maintain an erection is natural as we age. If at 20 we're ready to make love all night long, at 40 things can get a bit more complicated.

Various physical pathologies, which we'll look at shortly, can combine with psychological factors. Quite often, one or two "duds" can suffice to be assailed by doubts and a tremendous performance anxiety. We thus find ourselves in a spiral of stress and worry, the main enemies of sexual serenity.

Now, to those sexual partners who witness the penis's "deflation": what do you do? There are only a few rules: don't laugh, don't ever laugh; don't try to joke about the matter, not even just to downplay it; and don't feel responsible. It's necessary, however, to talk about it and be calm, trying to fantasize about the next opportunity. Trying again right away might not be a good idea. As with phimosis, erectile dysfunction can conceal more severe pathologies, which it's best to exclude before proceeding with a targeted therapy.

Let's look at some of them.

Endocrine pathologies. Diseases linked to hormonal alterations, such as hypogonadism, which occurs when a man's testosterone production rates begin to fall below the standard threshold. **Consequences of an operation in the abdominal or pelvic region**. An operation in these areas can damage the nerves that regulate the erection mechanism; sometimes these are cut accidentally, or for clinical reasons, as in the case of prostate cancer surgery.

Alterations in the cardio-circulatory system. A heart attack, arterial hypertension, a blood clot or thrombosis alter the functioning of the whole mechanism regulating erection. Consider, too, that taking drugs for high blood pressure can generate side effects.

Clinical studies also suggest that erectile dysfunction can appear shortly before a cardio-circulatory problem, typically a heart attack. This occurs because the penis is formed by a multiplicity of blood vessels smaller than those of the heart and, since a heart attack is merely the obstruction of a vessel, such blockages frequently appear first in the penis.

Taking NSAIDs. NSAIDs are nonsteroidal anti-inflammatory drugs, commonly used to combat fever, pain and inflammation (Naproxen, Acetylsalicylic Acid, Ibuprofen, and Ketoprofen are the most widespread). For some men, taking these drugs regularly makes erectile dysfunction 1.4 times more likely.

Diabetes. At least half the patients affected by diabetes experience an erectile insufficiency. This depends on the damage caused by diabetes to certain tissues, both at an arterial and neurological level. The excess glucose in the blood damages the penis's microvascular structures, bonding with the vessel walls and the tissues' structural proteins, making them less elastic and less inclined to dilate to allow the influx of blood necessary for an erection.

With so many causes of erectile dysfunction, following a diagnostic protocol is crucial.

This begins with a thorough anamnesis—gathering the data of the patient's personal history as they've experienced it. To this end we use the **International Index of Erectile Function—IIEF 5**, which evaluates erectile functioning in the last six months simply and specifically.

Try to answer as honestly as possible.

Each question contains 5 possible answers, with a score from 0 to 5. Choose and circle only one of them: the answer 0 means a complete absence of sexual activity.

The lower the score, the more significant the problem.

Before beginning, keep in mind that by "sexual activity" we mean intercourse, touching, foreplay and masturbation, by "intercourse" penetration, and by "sexual stimulation" situations like foreplay with a partner, looking at erotic images, etc. "Ejaculation" is defined as expulsion of sperm from the penis (or the feeling of doing so).

1) In the last six months, how would you rate your ability to reach and maintain an erection?

    0—practically non-existent
    1—very low
    2—low
    3—moderate
    4—high
    5—very high

2) In the last six months, after sexual stimulation, how often have you reached an erection sufficient for penetration?

    0—no sexual activity
    1—almost never or never
    2—not very often (much less than half the time)
    3—sometimes (roughly half the time)
    4—most of the time (much more than half the time)
    5—almost always or always

3) In the last six months, during intercourse, how often have you been able to maintain an erection after penetration?

    0—I didn't try to have intercourse
    1—almost never or never
    2—not very often (much less than half the time)
    3—sometimes (roughly half the time)
    4—most of the time (much more than half the time)
    5—almost always or always

4) In the last six months, during intercourse, how difficult has it been to maintain an erection until the end
of intercourse?

    0—I didn't try to have intercourse
    1—extremely difficult
    2—very difficult
    3—difficult
    4—relatively easy
    5—easy

5) In the last six months, during intercourse, how often
have you felt pleasure?

    0—I haven't tried to have intercourse
    1—almost never or never
    2—not very often (much less than half the time)
    3—sometimes (roughly half the time)
    4—most of the time (more than half the time)
    5—almost always or always

Calculate Your Score:
Severe Erectile Dysfunction: from 5 to 7
Moderate Erectile Dysfunction: from 8 to 11
Slight-to-Moderate Erectile Dysfunction: from 12 to 16
Slight Erectile Dysfunction: from 17 to 21
No Erectile Dysfunction: from 22 to 25

A Matter of Reputation

Florence is divided into four historic quarters, each characterized by a specific color. Every June 24, the day the city celebrates

its patron saint, John the Baptist, Piazza Santa Croce turns into a field for Historic Florentine Football. Four teams, one representing each quarter, face off against one another to commemorate, per the tradition, the first match on February 17, 1530, played during the siege of the city by Charles V's Spanish troops.

Marco is thirty-three years old and single. He's a man that anyone would define as "good-looking." In Florence everybody knows him because he's a historic football player; all his friends consider him a playboy, someone who has no shortage of opportunities to sleep with women. Yet for six months, he hasn't been able to have an erection that allows him to conclude intercourse in a satisfying manner.

A few days after the tournament, I see him in my office in the heart of Florence. Even though I recognize him, I pretend I don't to avoid embarrassing him.

He tells me that his life has gone to pieces: while he used to go out with a different girl every night, now he's shut up at home with only Netflix to keep him company. It all began after meeting an American girl much younger than him. The night he spent with her was, in his words, tragic.

"Doc, my dick got *barzotto*, but then it couldn't go any further. I was concerned, but not excessively because, well, it happens to everyone. But a few days later I tried again with a gorgeous Swedish girl—you know, Florence is a really popular destination for Erasmus students . . . If you're wondering why I prefer foreigners to Italian girls, it's because if someone gabs, I'm ruined. My reputation precedes me!"

Note for non-Florentines: "*barzotto*" is a quite un-scientific expression for when the penis is only partially erect.

Marco isn't on any medication, he doesn't smoke or do drugs, he drinks red wine with meals and some harder liquors on occasion. The examination doesn't show anything out of the ordinary:

he does tell me that lately, after training sessions, he's been feeling strange, very tired; but then he corrects himself—the sessions are very demanding and, all things considered, it's normal.

I wonder if there's a psychological problem that Marco isn't mentioning. I put him at ease and prescribe a series of blood tests to run before deciding on a therapy thanks to which, I tell him, "Everything will go back to normal."

After several days Marco texts me that the tests have revealed an abnormal value, marked with an asterisk. I tell him to send them to me or come by the office.

He walks in less than 20 minutes later. His basal blood sugar level is 225 mg/dL, when the norm should be between 60 and 110: with a number like, the diagnosis is clearly diabetes. Marco is devastated. The first thing he blurts out is: "I won't be able to play anymore?"

I reassure him, explaining that diabetes is treatable and that he'll be able to continue practicing sports; in fact, physical activity will really help him. But most of all, I tell him to look at the upside: those "tragic" nights of his led him to discover a pathology which otherwise would have long remained hidden, only to manifest itself very seriously.

Now Marco is receiving treatment at a diabetes center and his blood sugar level is under control, his sex life has returned to normal, and his "honor," about which he was so worried, is intact.

The next step is to proceed with clinical-instrumental tests, particularly those of a hematic nature measuring blood sugar, cholesterol, and triglycerides. Then it's on to second-level diagnostics, including an echo color doppler (ECD).

Carefully selected cases then make recourse to the **RigiScan**, a device that analyzes whether or not there's a physiological component at the root of the problem. It registers unconscious nocturnal erections: if they occur, the system is functioning regularly; if they don't, further investigation is necessary.

After the diagnostic phase, we proceed to a therapeutic path to resolve the erectile dysfunction. The most suitable solution changes from one patient to another because it's linked to personal habits and aspirations. Often, it's sufficient to explain the need to correct a series of mistaken habits concerning smoking, alcohol, drugs, or a sedentary lifestyle. Subsequently we can call on "first-line" therapeutic solutions, consisting in oral or intraurethral medications.

Second-line therapies, on the other hand, consist of injections or the use of devices, while surgery is a last resort or for the most serious cases.

First-Line Therapy for Erectile Dysfunction: Oral or Intra-Urethral Drugs

At this level we intervene with medication that's easy to take, in the form of pills or film that dissolves on the tongue. This category includes **inhibitors of phosphodiesterase type-5 (PDE5)**, an enzyme present in the corpora cavernosa's muscular cells. The medication relaxes the smooth muscle, encourages the influx of blood and consequently facilitates erection. This solution might seem quite chemical and not very romantic, but one of its winning aspects is that the active ingredient is only engaged in the presence of an erotic stimulus. The partner is thus essential for the treatment's success.

Four molecules are suitable for performing this task, and they induce very different effects: Sildenafil (or Viagra), which induces potency; Vardenafil (or Levitra), which induces speed; Tadalafil (or Cialis), which aids with continuity; and Avanafil (or Spedra), which boosts confidence.

It's a range that covers a broad spectrum of needs. There's no scale of priority; or better, no molecule is more correct than another. It isn't possible to give univocal indications without knowing the habits of the individual: the specialist will determine the most appropriate medication on a case-by-case basis, a customized therapy for the patient, like at the tailor's.

To "take the measurements," it's first necessary to investigate the patient's experience with medications and his frequency of sexual relations. A great deal depends in fact on the patient's expectations and those of his partner, who doesn't always want to have to deal with an unmanageable erection and may thus prefer a fast-acting drug of shorter duration, maintaining the naturalness of intercourse and eliminating the need for planning.

Drugs against erectile dysfunction generally don't cause adverse reactions and are effective, but no studies prove that one is any better than the others, though early on people thought that daily use brought about improvements in spontaneous erection. The only molecule currently suitable for daily use is Tadalafil 5 mg.

The factors that should orient a urologist's choice to one active ingredient or another are age, sexual habits, time of day in which the patient usually has intercourse, interactions with other medications, and food and alcohol consumption.

I want to underline here that there is a sex life beyond erectile dysfunction, and let it be clear that this includes auto-eroticism. The turning point came in the late 1990s with the formulation of Viagra, which is simply the commercial name of Sildenafil. It arrived in Italy on March 27, 1998: I clearly remember that day because on the tenth anniversary of its introduction I wrote an editorial in a famous daily newspaper. This molecule had provoked enormous interest in the scientific community and, with perhaps even greater clamor, among everyday citizens. It was a landmark, similar to what had happened 20 years earlier with the birth control pill for women. People thought that this magic pill could solve any problem. The manufacturer turned it into a symbol, adopting the blue pill as its logo, proudly and unequivocally laying claim to its creation. With Viagra we can re-establish a now-lost sexual activity in 80% of cases. It was a true turning point, leading multiple generations to conclude that the idea of sexuality as linked to reproduction was definitively shelved. Culturally, it was a genuine revolution. In all honesty, today we can state that, thanks to medicine and surgery, perhaps combined, no male patient without particularly serious physical complications is incapable of having a satisfying, even an excellent sex life.

Like any drugs, Viagra has side effects, but they're limited. At the time of the blue pill's appearance on the market, several reactions appeared and they were broadly amplified in the media, with the aim of generating anxiety. You would've thought it had killed one user after another. In truth there were very few deaths, not only in absolute terms but also in relation to the total number of patients treated, and the cause wasn't even the drug, but rather age and physical condition. To use a comparison, it isn't reasonable to send out an eighty-year-old, least of all one devoid of any training, to run a 100-meter dash: if he has a heart attack and dies during or after the race, you wouldn't say the race itself was the cause. In the same way, if thanks to Viagra an eighty-year-old resumes sexual activity, perhaps after a ten or 20-year hiatus, and does so at an intense pace, he's subjecting himself to significant physical strain that might even be fatal.

Fortunately, over time we have figured out how to "calibrate" therapy and behaviors, and today even cardiologists prescribe these drugs. To simplify, they are vasodilators, discovered, what's more, entirely by chance. Researchers were searching for vasodilators that were better than nitro derivatives—quite powerful, yet quite limited in terms of duration—and they realized that although the Viagra molecule induced a mild result, patients reported improved sexual activity. Like Christopher Columbus, who landed in America while searching for the Indies, these modern-day explorers discovered the pharmacological El Dorado while navigating in a different direction.

Meriting a separate discussion, on the other hand, is the risk posed by the illegal sale of these drugs. Many a website offers the chance to purchase Viagra, Levitra, Cialis and the like without a medical prescription, but this is prohibited in Italy, even when the drugs come from other countries, and constitutes a criminal offense. Such websites, furthermore, provide no guarantee of what you'll receive at home. Several years ago, an investigative pool of medical specialists and law enforcement experts purchased an online sampling of these products: 50% of the time no package arrived (online fraud, pure and simple), while in the other 50% the product was a placebo. From a medical standpoint, better nothing than a harmful product: in many of the pseudo-drugs investigators found traces of nitrates and other prohibited harmful substances. Purchasing medication through non-official channels exposes buyers to high risks of economic loss and, sometimes, even a danger to one's health.

Like the other PDE5 inhibitors, Viagra should not be purchased online and before using it you should talk to a doctor. But the perception, from the external standpoint of the illegal market, is that there is a great deal of it in circulation, even when not medically required. It's undeniable that it's used recreationally, more or less at all ages, for a one-off exceptional performance. Data reveal that 50% of the time it's used "just for fun." Meaning tens of millions of doses each year.

20 years ago I convinced a group of urology residents to participate in a study to evaluate the consequences of taking Viagra for men aged 25–30 without erectile dysfunction. I used the

drug along with a placebo and proceeded blindly, meaning the participants didn't know which of the two they were taking. The experiment showed that the erection they achieved was normal, but what changed was merely the refractory period, or the time interval between one session of intercourse and the next. In young men, for whom the interval is already brief, it was eliminated altogether. The exercise was also useful for understanding that for men 25–30 the drug is useless, while in men 40–45 it's useful for impressing someone, but it doesn't protect you from the risks. We must always remember that any drug requires a prior medical examination and therapeutic indication from your doctor.

Another drug that has appeared recently is a **prostaglandin specifically for erection**. It's as a single-dose liquid medication to be inserted, if necessary, into the urethra, relaxing certain muscles in the penis through the dilation of several blood vessels.

Patients with circulatory issues can also consider the use of **shock waves**, analogous to the high-intensity waves used to break up kidney stones. In this case, the mechanism consists of using waves—of low intensity in this case—to stimulate angiogenesis, or the production of new blood vessels.

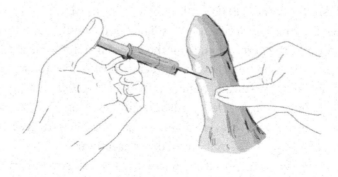

Figure n. 20—Prostaglandin injection

Second-Line Therapy for Erectile Dysfunction: Relatively Invasive Drugs

If the arsenal available up to this point doesn't give the desired response, we proceed to second-line solutions, composed of slightly more invasive treatments. We can use what patients refer to as "shots," penile injections containing **prostaglandin**. The active ingredient, similar to that in liquid eye drops, is based on the drug's strength as a vasodilator and functions independently of erotic stimulus.

The operation is more complex than taking a drug, is generally painful, and requires good dexterity. It's also crucial to respect the dosage and be trained with a specialist to avoid unpleasant consequences, ranging from slight embarrassment to the need for immediate hospitalization, as when the injection causes **priapism**—a prolonged erection preventing the penis from returning to flaccidity.

For the most serious dysfunctions, the drug can be combined with a **penis pump**. This is a vacuum constriction machine that uses suction to create a vacuum and thus recalls blood to the penis, favoring erection. The pump has the advantage of not requiring an invasive operation, but its effects are less effective than implants. The pump is thus more suitable for men who are capable of achieving at least a partial erection on their own. A certain amount of preparation time is also required, so you'll have to forego spontaneity, at least in part. This device is also highly recommended for men who can't take drugs because it is purely mechanical in nature.

Third-Line Therapy for Erectile Dysfunction: The Surgical Option

Should both the first and second line fail to work, the next step is surgery. This calls for the insertion of a penile implant that permits a "controlled" erection.

I've positioned implants of this sort in boys of 18 and patients of 80. In all likelihood, partners won't notice anything new. **Penile implants** are composed of two cylinders inserted in the penis's corpora cavernosa, connected via little tubes to a reservoir of saline solution that is embedded beneath the rectal muscles in the lower abdomen. A pump is connected to the system and located beneath the soft skin of the scrotum, between the testicles. To inflate the prosthesis you press on the pump that transfers the saline solution from the reservoir to the cylinders in the penis, inflating them and provoking an erection. By pressing on a deflation valve at the base of the pump, the fluid returns to the reservoir, bringing the penis back to its normal flaccid state.

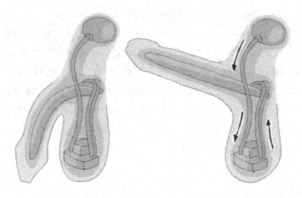

Figure n. 21—Penile implant

The prosthesis enables an erection that has a natural appearance. Most men with an implant judge their erection to be slightly shorter than normal, but the sensation on the skin of the penis and the ability to reach orgasm are practically unchanged. Ejaculation isn't negatively influenced.

After the insertion of a prosthesis, it's no longer possible to have a spontaneous erection. Should the implant have to be removed, the man can no longer have natural erections. This shouldn't represent a problem, however, given that if this operation is necessary such capacity has already been compromised.

Premature Ejaculation

We now move on to another aspect of sexuality. In the medical field **premature ejaculation** refers to when the duration of intercourse, due to the man's orgasm, lasts less than one minute. The reason for the cessation, however, must be connected to an inability to delay the sexual response voluntarily: this is the discriminating factor. Most men are able to delay orgasm, simply put, to "hold back" for a certain period of time; those who suffer from premature ejaculation cannot. We aren't talking about so-called "quickies," which are actually quite healthy for a couple and testify to mutual desire even when time is short, especially when there are children involved.

The official data indicate that the phenomenon of premature ejaculation affects 20% of young men, but I honestly don't think so. If anything, this could be true only in reference to patients who undergo urological examinations. In this case, yes, 20% of those who see a urologist do so for a problem of premature ejaculation. So the target no longer corresponds to 20% of the total population, but 20% of the patients who visit uro-andrology clinics, which is certainly a more truthful picture.

Accurate studies conducted in Turkey provide even more precise data. In the healthy population, premature ejaculation appears to affect only 3–4% of men. Personally I'm convinced that the real amount is even lower. We often forget that man is fundamentally an animal, with innate instincts that include reproduction. Ultimately, all animal species suffer from premature ejaculation: the lion mates quickly with the lioness because he could be disturbed by a competitor or a hunter; the same is true for a gazelle or a rabbit. On our evolutionary journey we have reserved an ever increasing space for the pursuit of pleasure, distancing ourselves further from the view of sex as merely for reproductive purposes. From this, perhaps, arises the vision of premature ejaculation as a disease, an opportunity which the pharmaceutical industry certainly to take advantage of. But the reality is quite different.

Clinically, only about 10% of patients who complain of premature ejaculation suffer from another pathology, such as hypothyroidism or prostatitis. The remaining 90% have no fundamental pathology.

In my experience, using drugs to treat anxiety is effective in postponing ejaculation. It isn't exactly a cure, but an attempt to help the patient who, for his part, should look into the deeper reasons for his situation, perhaps with the help of a therapist.

How else can the question be resolved? Patients often tell me that they've practiced distracting themselves during sex: memorizing the seven kings of ancient Rome, Italy's lineup at the last World Cup, the ingredients for Spaghetti all'Amatriciana, or the following day's work schedule. For those who suffer from premature ejaculation, this isn't possible.

Talking things over your partner is a necessary step, before investigating the question further with a specialist. Taking the time to talk and trying to pleasure one another in other ways not exclusively aimed at penetration is important, because sex isn't a competition. The mutual exploration of pleasure, foreplay and natural stimulation can ease preoccupations.

I'm convinced that many problems can be resolved by dialogue, improving our knowledge of our body, and perhaps by following well-founded, traditional advice such as making recourse to masturbation, even as adults and, possibly, before meeting our partner.

Dialogue with the patient, understanding his needs, is the first therapeutic step: these are points on which I always insist. In medicine today we speak of a "patient-centered" visit, or "counseling." It's a fundamental approach for acquiring information about his life, his discomfort and its origins. Researchers claim that it takes a specialist an average of eighteen seconds to gain a clear picture of the situation; I think that with one minute more you can reach a truly precise diagnosis, even if experts usually speak of at least 20–30 minutes. It's a subjective datum: sometimes I can be very quick, despite dedicating the maximum care to evaluating the patient's experience. As far as the sphere of sexual pathologies is concerned—and the problem of premature ejaculation in particular—this point is fundamental.

If the problem of premature ejaculation persists even after such a consultation, perhaps combined with counseling from a psychosexual therapist, we can look at other therapeutic options: **Dapoxetine**, for example. Several years ago I dedicated an essay to this topic, and the title pretty much says it all: "Dapoxetine: The Reasons for a Waterloo." Its level of effectiveness is good— in 60% of cases the duration of intercourse triples. It's also easily to manage, since it's taken orally 1–3 hours prior to intercourse. The point, however, is that it induces rather serious side effects, including nausea, diarrhea, headache, addiction, and what in medicine is called the "drop-out effect," or negative effects at therapy's end.

Prior to its use, on the other hand, the side effects that certain psychiatric drugs induced in time before ejaculation was exploited. Among these were **SSRI antidepressants or clomipramines**, which today continue to be used in an off-label regime, meaning that the therapeutic effect isn't expressly mentioned in the packaged instructions. Yet such drugs demand extreme prudence due to their risk—very low, but still present—of inducing self-harm, even suicide.

There are also local anesthetics, including a specific compound of **lidocaine** and **prilocaine**, distributed in spray form and used five minutes prior to intercourse. It prolongs time before ejaculation by an average of 6 times, with reduced side effects including anesthesia of the genitals, experienced by 4.5% of men and 1% of their partners.

Lastly, you can turn to several devices, similar to bandages, applied to the perineum. Via electrical impulses, they can improve ejaculation time and might soon represent an easy solution to this unpleasant anomaly.

An Engineer Isn't a Urologist

This is the short story of Fabrizio, an engineer of thirty with a brilliant university career, a well-paying job and a passion for DIY. He diagnosed himself with premature ejaculation, of which none of his partners had ever complained: neither the few women he slept with in his younger years nor the men he sees now.

After doing some research on the topic he discovers on Google that for many years it was thought that premature ejaculation could be resolved by circumcision. The reasoning was the following: the removal of the foreskin causes the loss of the nerve endings connected to it and causes the glans to dry out, reducing sensitivity and thus prolonging intercourse.

Today everyone knows that this isn't the case.

First of all, a proper surgical circumcision causes no mutilation whatsoever; secondly, recent studies conducted on thousands of cases have thoroughly proven that circumcision doesn't influence ejaculation time. Circumcised males have no greater or lesser probability of suffering from premature ejaculation, or feeling more or less pleasure—or pain—during intercourse.

But Fabrizio convinces himself of it, partly because he believes his abundant foreskin is somehow responsible for the dysfunction, and he sets to building an artisanal circumcision apparatus. He's too embarrassed to turn to a medical clinic and he thinks that his futile motives don't justify the cost of seeing a specialist. In addition, he trusts in his manual skills.

Our paths cross just forty-eight hours after his endeavor.

"Nicola, you need to come to the ER immediately," says Lucia, a colleague of mine, on the phone.

"We have a guy with a necrosis of the glans. I've never seen anything like it! Prepare yourself, you won't believe your eyes!"

I get dressed, still half asleep, and leave for the hospital. After talking with the engineer, who's quite calm despite the situation, I discover his plan: "I thought that by going through the National Health Service I would have to wait months, and when the moment finally came I would be mocked due to the reason I wanted to be circumcised."

"Which is?"

"Prolonging my erection time. Seeing a specialist privately, on the other hand, would have required too much money."

I stare at him, speechless.

After recovering my wits, I explain that there's no medical correlation between circumcision and the solution to premature ejaculation. I have him tell me exactly what he did to his penis. As Lucia had warned me, I can't believe my eyes. "I took the cap of a bottle of water, perforated the flat part and kept only the outer ring. I lowered my foreskin, inserted this ring, and pulled the skin back up. I waited for forty-eight hours and what was supposed to be a necrosis that would have detached the excess part was created. But this didn't happen, so here I am."

I imagine that he didn't minimally take into consideration that such operations must be done by expert hands, in a sterile environment.

"We need to go straight to the operating room."

If it isn't caught in time, a necrosis of this magnitude can necessitate a partial or even a total amputation of the penis. Fortunately we're able to remove the now-compromised section, then partially reconstruct the foreskin.

After waking up from the anesthesia, Fabrizio thanks us. In a month's time, his penis will regain its normal appearance.

On my check-up rounds a few hours later, I stick my head in his room.

"Sir, a piece of advice: in life, always remember that 'the more you spend, the less you spend.' DIY solutions aren't always the best ones! And when you have a chance, see me at my clinic, we'll do a serious evaluation of your ejaculation."

There are other problems linked to ejaculation that deserve a closer look.

Delayed ejaculation, for example. It's a medical or psychological condition that occurs when you don't feel the need to ejaculate or you feel it after a very long time. A specialist visit can identify the causes and an ad hoc solution. Among the medical causes we have antidepressants, high blood pressure medications or antipsychotic drugs, incomplete spinal lesions, or pathologies linked to the prostate. At present we do not possess an approved, specifically-indicated drug. A generic suggestion dictated by experience that I would give is to reduce masturbation and see if the condition improves.

We also have **retrograde ejaculation**. In this case the patient reaches orgasm but doesn't ejaculate, because the sperm ends up in the bladder. This is a delicate situation that can conceal the onset of diabetes or be the consequence of certain operations that regard the genital area, such as those to cure a benign prostatic hypertrophy. It sometimes happens that urologists, in the pre-operation phase, forget to inform the patient of this unpleasant follow-up, allowing the frustration and discomfort to appear in all their force in the post-surgery phase. But the condition can also have a pharmacological genesis. It can be caused, for example, by alphalitics, used to manage the symptoms of prostatitis. By identifying the precise cause, and related corrective action, the problem is quickly resolved. If not, it can even become permanent.

In **painful ejaculation** the burning that you feel after ejaculating is localized between the penis, scrotum and perineum. Many can be the causes, beginning with idiopathic forms—those with unclear origins—and ranging to infections of the region between the prostate, testicles and urethra. Therapies include specific drugs or radiotherapy. If the symptom doesn't appear with ejaculation, the psychological component should also be considered.

Then there's **anejaculation**, or the condition of total absence of ejaculation, neither externally nor in the bladder, even when you orgasm. It typically occurs in patients operated for cancer with the removal of the prostate and seminal vesicles. In general, in fact, the problem is linked to surgical operations, medication or a syndrome of the urogenital region. It certainly shouldn't be underestimated, opting for an always opportune specialist visit.

As the alpha privative teaches, **anorgasmia**, on the other hand, is the absence of orgasm, often associated with the absence of ejaculation but also experienced in its presence. It should in no way be confused with infertility or erectile dysfunction: it can be congenital—present from birth—or arise suddenly in the course of life, due to a fall in testosterone or the use of psychiatric or illegal drugs, or even have an origin of a psychological nature.

Finally we have **hematospermia**: that situation in which in the semen there are traces of blood. Its cause is generally identifiable in an infection of the genital apparatus—the prostate, for example—or in certain antiplatelet drugs, but you cannot exclude the possibility—even if rare—of looking at a tumoral form.

My advice is to make an urgent appointment to clarify the true state of things.

Peyronie's Disease

Let's return to the age/state of health duo. We know by now that diseases with consequences on the health of the penis can arise at any age, but it is certainly true that adulthood covers a long part of an individual's life, so it's statistically frequent that specific pathologies appear in this period.

Peyronie's disease (or Induratio Penis Plastica) gets its name from Monsieur La Peyronie, a French doctor who served at the court of Louis XV who described it in detail because he suffered from it. It's considered rare, even if in truth it isn't that uncommon, since it affects between 5–7% of men over fifty, reaching almost 10% in certain contexts.

In the literature it's described beginning with three symptoms: penile curvature, pain (sometimes intense), erectile problems. The first true early symptom is penile pain, which increases exponentially during erection. It's caused by a sort of plaque present on the shaft, whose presence the patient doesn't notice for several days or even months. Appearing at this point can be a deformity, in this case a curvature (patients usually call it "crookedness") with angles ranging from 10 to 90 or more degrees. In certain cases it can even appear with shrinkage of the circumference, giving the shaft an hourglass shape. Over time, it also causes a quite visible shortening of the penis. If there are other concurrent pathologies—diabetes, hypertension or conditions of a psychological nature—there will also be erectile problems.

The disease includes two phases: the first, which is defined "active," is inflammatory in nature. It covers an average interval of roughly 9–12 months, increasing in some cases to as many as 18. Then follows a pause of stabilization which precedes the terminal phase, chronic or fibrotic. The cause is still unknown to this day. Until recently it was thought that the disease could be triggered by repeated microtraumas, but today the genetic hypothesis has gained ground, supported by data that indicate that 30% of those who suffer from it have a father or brother who does as well. I favor this interpretive line, given that in my clinical experience I have treated fifteen-year-old virgin patients affected by the disease.

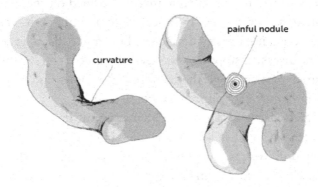

Figure n. 22—Peyronie's Disease

The diagnosis is quite simple, made via a simple examination of the penis. The expert specialist is quickly able to identify the "pebbles," similar to plaques, which form on the inside of the shaft, but to be certain an echo color doppler is useful. An ultrasound, in fact, makes it possible to highlight the morphology and vascularization of the penis, as well as to understand if we're in the active phase or the pause of stabilization. In the first case, the patient will be facing several months in which he will see the situation worsen, in the second he will know that the maximum amount of damage has been done. At most, he might see a further shortening of the penis.

Until a few years ago, we didn't know much about Peyronie's Disease—I'd go as far as to say that we knew next to nothing—we made recourse to palliative treatments and waited for it to run its course. Even today, supplements and exercises are prescribed for the purpose of stabilizing the patient's conditions. Luckily things have evolved.

In the United States first and then in Europe, in 2013 and 2015 respectively, there appeared a targeted drug based on *Clostridium Histolyticum* collagenase. This is an enzyme that, when inserted into the plaque that has formed on the penis, is able to attack it, literally to "eat it" by modifying it. Over time the plaque doesn't disappear, but rather disintegrates, and the disease is stopped. If it's treated quickly, you can even be cured, particularly if the damage isn't serious, and by and large curvature can improve by 20–30 degrees.

A great deal of fake news circulate about this drug, one of which says that it leads to penile rupture. This has only occurred in five cases worldwide. As for the cases that I have personally treated, in only two: the first at three weeks from the treatment, the second in the days immediately following and caused by the failure to observe the rules accompanying the treatment, including exercises.

I have been something of a pioneer when it comes to Peyronie's Disease, because I was the first in Italy to use this collagenase-based drug. Today, with over a thousand patients treated, I have treated the most clinical cases of anyone in the world. 80% of the patients who follow the pharmacological therapy say that they are satisfied upon its conclusion. This is a truly encouraging result, partly because the pathology is seriously incapacitating, to the point of not permitting sexual relations. The fact is, I consider it more of a couple's disease than an individual's, because the partner is a victim of it as well.

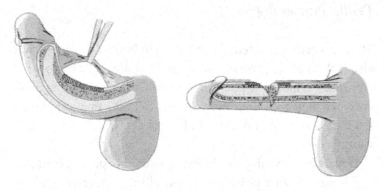

Figure n. 23—Peyronie's Disease plaque removal operation

An 80% cure rate should be considered an excellent result. For the other 20%, it is still possible to consider undertaking a surgical solution. To decide, you should first of all ask yourself whether or not you're capable of having sexual activity. If the answer is yes, you can decide to leave things as they are. Vice versa, if the pathology is so incapacitating that it prevents it, you can decide to opt for surgery. In this last case, however, a problem arises. Regardless of the technical solution adopted, there will be a price to pay in terms of modification of the penis.

With simple surgery, meaning operating from the long side, it's possible to straighten it but there is an inevitable shortening of 1–2 centimeters. If, however, you extract the plaque from the short side, the penis is straightened and a sort of "patch" is inserted, composed of human material (a vein or other tissue) or heterologous, synthetic or from bovine samples. In this case a part of the corpora cavernosa is eliminated as well and the erectile mechanism is damaged. The risk of this approach, therefore, is generating impotence, which must be resolved with a further operation to position a penis implant.

Penile Shortening

The penis can be shortened not only with Peyronie's Disease but also with a radical prostatectomy, in the context of a removal of a prostatic tumor. The phenomenon can also occur in the presence of a metabolic condition. In this case, the man registers a fall in testosterone and a rise in fat mass, in which the penis is subsumed.

If there aren't visible modifications but only pain, it could be a phlebitis—a state of inflammation of the surface vein of the penis. Technically this is **Penile Mondor's Disease**, similar to a condition of varicose veins in a woman.

Its appearance can be determined by "overuse of the penis," or excessive masturbation. The therapy is simple and consists of sexual repose: the solution appears in a few days, though the feeling of pain can continue for several months.

Another cause can lead us to a penile microtrauma, but the pain disappears on its own within a few hours. It could also be **urethritis,** or an infection or inflammation within the urethra.

Here the pain appears almost exclusively during urination, and it's treated with antibiotics. Lastly there are idiopathic cases as well, corresponding to situations in which, frankly, the causes and dynamics are completely unknown and they remain so. Fortunately in all these cases the pain ceases in precisely the same way it appears.

Prostatitis

As we've observed in the section dedicated to upkeep, one of the organs most at risk in the urogenital system in men between 30 and 40 is certainly the prostate. So let's discuss the variants of prostatitis.

The symptoms are various and can include pain in the perianal zone and testicles, difficulty urinating, burning, and pain in the lower abdomen. In all these cases the diagnosis is exclusively clinical. First of all it's necessary to figure out the outlines of the condition, conduct blood culture and swab tests to verify whether there is a bacterial or abacterial infection underway and, naturally, talk with the patient.

Prepared specifically for this purpose is the **NIH-CPSI questionnaire**: it doesn't serve to diagnose prostatitis, but to understand whether there's room for improvement with simple pharmacological protocols.

The form was developed in the United States and validated in Italy but a dear colleague of mine, Dr. Gianluca Giubilei.

A. *Pain or Discomfort*
   1) In the last week, have you had pain or discomfort in the following areas?
      a. Area between the anus and testicles (perineum)— yes (1 point) / no (0 points)

    b. Testicles—yes (1 point) / no (0 points)

    c. Tip of the penis (not when you urinate)—yes (1 point) / no (0 points)

    d. Below your waist, in the pubic zone or the bladder—yes (1 point) / no (0 points)

2) In the last week, have you had:

    a. Pain or burning when you urinate?—yes (1 point) / no (0 points)

    b. Pain or discomfort during or after orgasm (ejaculation)?—yes (1 point) / no (0 points)

3) In the last week, how many times have you had pain or discomfort in the aforementioned areas?

    a. Never (0 points)

    b. Rarely (1 point)

    c. Sometimes (2 points)

    d. Often (3 points)

    e. Usually (4 points)

    f. Always (5 points)

4) In the last week, what number best describes the average pain or discomfort on the days you felt it?

    1 2 3 4 5 6 7 8 9 10*

    10* is the worst pain imaginable

    The pain's numerical value is added to the score from the *Pain or Discomfort* category

B. Urination (urinary symptoms)

5) How many times in the last week have you felt like you didn't completely empty your bladder after urinating?

a. Never (0 points)

b. Less than one out of every five times (1 point)

c. Less than half the time (2 points)

d. Roughly half the time (3 points)

e. More than half the time (4 points)

f. Almost always (5 points)

6) In the last week, how many times have you had to urinate again less than two hours from the previous time?

a. Never (0 points)

b. Less than one out of every five times (1 point)

c. Less than half the time (2 points)

d. Roughly half the time (3 points)

e. More than half the time (4 points)

f. Almost always (5 points)

C. *Quality of Life (impact of symptoms on quality of life)*

7) In the last week, to what degree have the symptoms limited your daily activities?

a. Not at all (0 points)

b. Not much (1 point)

c. To some degree (2 points)

d. A lot (3 points)

8) How much have you thought about your symptoms in the last week?

a. Not at all (0 points)

b. Not much (1 point)

c. To some degree (2 points)

d. A lot (3 points)

9) If you had to spend the rest of your life with the symptoms of the last week, how would you feel?
    a. Quite satisfied (0 points)
    b. Satisfied (1 point)
    c. Moderately satisfied (2 points)
    d. Indifferent (3 points)
    e. Moderately unsatisfied (4 points)
    f. Unsatisfied (5 points)
    g. Terribly unsatisfied (6 points)

Calculate Your Score:

A. *Pain or Discomfort*
    Sum of questions 1a, 1b, 1c, 1d, 2a, 2b, 3, and 4
    =_____

B. *Urination (Urinary symptoms)*
    Sum of questions 5 and 6 =_____

C. *Quality of Life*
    Sum of questions 7, 8 and 9 =_____

Your NIH-CPSI Score
    The total of the three sums =_____

Your Symptoms
Sum of the *Pain and Discomfort* and *Urination* scores
    =_____

    Slight Symptomology: from 0 to 9
    Moderate Symptomology: from 10 to 18
    Severe Symptomology: from 19 to 31

You Wanted the Bicycle?

Alberto is forty-three, he's always been passionate about sports and after getting his degree in Sports Science he began teaching at the scientific high school in his town. He can never seem to get enough physical activity: two evenings a week he coaches a women's basketball team and, off and on, especially early in the season, he's the athletic trainer for a youth soccer team.

But his true passion is cycling. Even in winter he always goes out for a Sunday ride, with friends or alone: it can last up to five hours and is largely uphill.

He comes to the clinic because for some weeks now he's been feeling an unusual pain in the area below his testicles and retro-pubic area, so his wife, sick of hearing his complaints, has sent him to see me, since I've treated her best friend's husband. After discussing his symptoms and asking about his habits, I proceed with a rectal exploration. What emerges is a soft and extremely warm prostate, two factors that make me think of prostatitis.

Alberto is very concerned because he thinks that the cause is attributable to the many hours spent on his bike, but he isn't ready to give it up. But I explain it only needs to be set aside for a brief period, until he's completely healed.

The correlation between cycling and the prostate has long been debated. Today we can say that the bicycle doesn't cause anything but, if there are risk factors and a predisposition, it represents the trigger. For cases of prostatitis in particular, the pressure of the pelvic floor area on the seat causes increases the inflammation, which can become quite painful.

A few weeks after the first consultation I see Alberto again, who with great difficulty has managed to keep away from his beloved two-wheeler and is on the mend. Our meeting doesn't remain a simple check-up, however, but turns into a long discussion of the world of cycling. Alberto has gathered a great deal of information and gives me a sort of lecture on all the equipment necessary to protect the prostate while biking, ready for when he can get back to pedaling.

First he shows me his new purchase: shorts with a reinforced crotch. Then he shows me the bicycle seat with a hole in it—he's very proud of it.

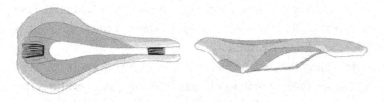

Figure n. 24—Bicycle seats for the pelvic floor

Professional seats with a central hole in the middle are ideal for the prostate, since the pressure is distributed on the sides, thus guaranteeing a correct weight distribution on the two ischial bones, leaving the perineal region free. For those who go on long bike rides, it can be a more than ideal solution.

When we say goodbye I thank him. Doctors can learn from their patients, too.

Cases of prostatitis caused by bacterial infection are resolved by simple antibiotics-based therapies. Even the acutest forms, with high fevers. Abacterial forms, on the other hand, are still obscure and are treated by modifying several aspects of your lifestyle. Sometimes with supplements, a diet with reduced amounts of certain foods—pepper, hot pepper, beer, white wine—and regular physical exercise.

Lastly, it's important to ejaculate frequently, because this act, whether alone or in company, helps more than a hundred drugs.

EMERGENCIES

In adulthood, penile traumas and ruptures are possible, if rare, events. What makes you wince is more the story that accompanies them, rather than the clinical aspect. A genital hematoma and the rupture of the penis are painful but easily resolved; much more complicated is saving the relationship, especially when the "crack" occurs outside of the domestic walls.

In addition to emergency care, on more than once occasion I've also provided assistance to the couple. Let's put it this way: a marriage is a worth a bandage. I'm sure that with all the archival material produced by my experience in the field, we could write a TV series complete with prequel, sequel and special episodes.

While penile rupture among adults is rare, even more so is **testicular torsion**. Common, on the other hand, is testicular infection, or **epididymitis**, which must be treated promptly to prevent it from degenerating into an abscess, with consequent loss of the testicle itself.

Even **cephalea** is a more common clinical circumstance than you might think—around age 20 and then between 35 and 45—and it can even appear during intercourse. It's characterized by a sudden and intense pain, which radiates from the base of the head to the nape and then the frontal part, affecting the temples and the occipital region. It is thought to be of a vasodilatory nature, connected, that is, to the increase in blood pressure near orgasm. It is usually benign, but it's always necessary to clarify its causes, particularly when associated with other symptoms like nausea, if it's protracted in time and occurs frequently. It could indicate an anomaly in a blood vessel, so it's a good idea to have an MRI. In rare cases it can be a precursor of serious cerebral pathologies.

I'm Not a Private Eye

Emanuele is thirty-eight and a doctor. But the reason he's at the ER isn't work-related, and it's clear from his visible agitation.

He has a large hematoma on his penis. To my colleague on call, Monica, he says that while he was playing tennis, he was serving and missed the ball, striking himself hard in the genital region. He's in intense pain.

Monica writes everything on his sheet but, as an ER veteran, she senses that something isn't right. Settings her doubts aside, she calls me, the on-call urologist, for the emergency.

When I arrive, I recognize Emanuele; in the last month we've discussed the pathologies of several patients and had lunch together a few times. He's just finished his residency.

"What are you doing here?"

"Nicola! I wasn't expecting to see you. Look, you'll never believe my bad luck . . ."

After listening to his story, I examine him and find a fractured penis. I express my doubts on the dynamics of the incident: the penis has to be erect to break.

"Hold on, Nicola, are you accusing me of lying? Don't you see how I'm dressed? I even have my tennis bag and racket at the front desk, where do you think I'm going? To the supermarket dressed in tennis clothes?"

Not to the supermarket, but quite possibly somewhere else. I see that he isn't calm and the fact that I insist on the likelihood of a rupture during intercourse makes him even more agitated. So I decide that for me, as a doctor, the objective evaluation of the situation is sufficient and that it's necessary to intervene immediately, avoiding further questions: the damage has been done, whether it was a racket or anything else.

The rupture (or fracture) of the penis occurs due to serious traumas of the penile shaft, particularly during sexual relations in which the partner is on top of the man. In statistical terms it's a rather rare event; in the scientific literature there were 1,500 cases in a period of almost 70 years (1935–2000).

As we saw in the last chapter, the laceration concerns the tunica albuginea that envelops the corpora cavernosa, with consequent and immediate pain, as well as the formation of a hematoma. Treatment must be prompt, with the application of ice and immediate hospitalization.

The diagnosis is confirmed by an examination and potential ultrasound and MRI, and the suggested therapy—the only one currently considered effective—is surgery.

In the operating room I proceed with the incision of the shaft to expose the damaged tissue, aspirating the local hematoma and finally recomposing the pieces via suture. In Emanuele's case the urethra, which would have required the insertion of a silicone catheter, wasn't harmed. After concluding this phase, I close up the incision.

Duration and typology of post-op recovery vary partly depending on how soon the operation occurs, which is why I decided to suspend my questioning. Full recovery, in any case, will require 6–12 weeks of rest. Emanuele's penis is safe and sound, it'll just have to take a little break. I meet Monica as she's finishing her shift. "You know that he wasn't telling you the truth, right?" she says. "There's no way that's how it happened."

"All's well that ends well. I'm not a private eye." Two years after the mysterious incident, I stop to chat in the hospital corridors. Gianfranco, informed as always about the latest ward gossip, can't resist giving me the day's scoop.

"Did you hear Emanuele's wife caught him cheating on her with an older woman? At the umpteenth evening tennis tournament, she got suspicious and found out she was right. Absurd." I pretend to be very surprised.

Post-coital cephalea, on the other hand, is usually related to the use of drugs that favor erection. When people suffer from this condition, the best advice is not to give in to anxiety and to try to relax. If the pain persists, it's good to get examined by a doctor and specify the drug in question. **Piercings**, too, can cause emergency situations. To begin with, they don't allow you to wear condoms securely. The foreign object, in fact, exponentially increases the chances of the condom breaking, so all sexual relations are high risk. Furthermore, they increase the chances of causing cuts in the vagina and anus.

They also risk creating fistulas in the penis. In this way the urine can take different channels, ending up no longer exiting the meatus but from another point along the shaft. This leads to a genuine and permanent lowering of the quality of life in the subject who suffers it, and possibly to a serious infection. So resist the idea and, if you simply must do it, rely only on competent medical personnel, always in conditions of total security.

What does it mean to be an adult? This is our incredibly vast query, which concerns such diverse fields that it could many more pages and many more books. What I can say is that it presumes a responsible attitude to one's own health and to that of those close to us. Having periodic checkups, encouraging family members to talk with specialists, teaching children the importance of medical science. This doesn't mean, of course, that the Batman costume needs to be locked up in the attic forever. I still wear mine quite proudly.

Dangerous Toys

Sofia and Simone have a very intense sex life that's free of preconceptions. They love telling each other their sexual fantasies and watching pornographic films together. But why just be spectators when they can play a starring role?

They decide to consult an online sex shop to realize their desires while maintaining their anonymity. Among their purchases is a steel cock ring, suggested to obtain a more intense, long-lasting erection through the sensation of the cold of the metal and, thanks to a decoration in relief, to stimulate Sofia's clitoris.

The ring is placed on the base of the penis but, as sometimes occurs with online purchases, the couple didn't calculate the correct measurements. The cock ring goes on, when Simone's penis has reached a semi-erect state, but then it won't come off.

The forced constriction blocks the outflow of blood and causes a situation similar to priapism: his penis is unable to return to its flaccid state and what begins as a game turns into a tragedy. After three hours and various attempts to remove the ring, they decide to get their courage up and go to the ER. I examine Simone immediately and I realize that the only way to free him is to find wire cutters. Not knowing who to turn to and given the late hour and lack of maintenance personnel in the vicinity, I decide to call the fire station without giving too much detail.

Within half an hour a fire truck brings me the tool. In the operating room we put the patient to sleep, in the hopes that the swelling of penis subsides to facilitate the cut, but this doesn't happen. The operation is very delicate: it's necessary to pop the ring off without compromising the shaft.

The cut is clean and precise. After freeing Simone, I heave a sigh of relief. His penis wasn't compromised and will be back to normal within a few days.

When I give the wire cutters back to a fireman waiting at the front desk, he says: "Doctor, tell him to take better measurements for the engagement ring, or else it'll be a real mess."

Even the walls in this hospital seem to have ears.

4

THE ELDERLY PENIS

"Marco, look who's come to pick you up today: Grandpa!"
"Actually, I'm his dad."

In 2018 the scientific community, and more specifically the Italian Society of Geronotology and Geriatrics (SIGG), modified the entrance threshold for elderhood from sixty-five to seventy-five years of age. With the increase in life expectancy of recent decades, people preferred to adopt a more precise classification with the generic definition of the "autumn of life."

In doing so we don't wish to mark the phases of life with a red pen, because categorizing individual experience is never a good idea. It's an indication that was as valid in adolescence as it is in this final chapter. Yet for effective communication it's always useful to delimit at least generally the audience to whom we're addressing our message.

We have thus decided to use SIGG's classification, partly because, in addition to at the social level, the problems that a man of sixty-eight encounters are different than those of an eighty-three-year-old in the medical field as well. And we're also in agreement on the fact that, today, considering a sixty-five-year-old as elderly is anachronistic.

To nuance the concept of old age we've identified four sub-groups: **young seniors** *(sixty-four to seventy-four years old),* **seniors** *(seventy-five to eighty-four years old),* **super seniors** *(eighty-five to ninety-nine years old) and* **centenarians.** *Comparing expectation and quality of life with those of thirty years ago, it seems excessively simple to state that the seventies are the new fifties!*

The following pages are thus destined to old age in its generic meaning, sure, but with the differentiations that we've just observed, even when they aren't directly specified.

Times change. Life expectancy has increased, as have the performances required of us by the outside world. Even retirement today is more distant and that age in which you were "just" (so to speak") a grandpa is full of potential.

I'll take the opportunity to say once and for all that **andropause** doesn't exist and has never existed. It's a decidedly abused term, not just by the media but also by doctors and health-sector professionals. Coined to emulate "menopause," which concludes a woman's ability to procreate, it has no reason to exist because for men it's a situation that never crops up. There is no "pause" in the production of sperm, which actually continues into old age, nor in the ability to fertilize a uterus, as long as the latter isn't on "pause."

This is why Marco's father, the man from this chapter's initial scene, was confused with a grandpa. To him I would suggest joining my personal battle, arming himself with a good sense of humor and perhaps a t-shirt that reads "Andropause is fake news and I'm living proof of it." Nevertheless, even if the spirit remains youthful, our body ages and undergoes changes for which we need to be prepared, to understand them and accept them. And this is precisely where urologists once again come into play.

So we come to old age. Before delving into the details of this final chapter, a warning: during this period of time the real trap to avoid is giving in to the fear of aging, of no longer being attractive and, consequently, of abandoning our sexuality.

UPKEEP

As we get up there in years our body bears and undergoes the process of aging: our back hunches over, our strength and stamina aren't what they once were, and nor is our hearing. The penis certainly isn't exempt from these changes: the skin that covers it begins to lose its elasticity and its color changes. The lesser blood supply produces less intense tones, particularly in the glans, and the natural fall in the testosterone rate causes pubic hair to become sparser.

Some websites claim that, past a certain age, the penis begins to shorten, losing up to 1 centimeter per year. I'd like to clear the field immediately of this fake news. Among other things, on those same sites are publicized and sold creams, pills, balms and other miraculous concoctions, which are supposedly capable of stopping the alleged shrinking process and maybe even reverse it. They are all quack remedies that in the best of cases are useless (if they are ever delivered to those who order them). The question is devoid of any medical or scientific foundation.

The phantom theory probably originated in the statistics on cases of dysmorphophobia, and particularly of penile curvature. It is hypothesized, indeed, that a rarer use of the organ and lesser quantity of erections cause, like for an athlete who stops running, the muscles to withdraw, thus favoring this curvature. Such a phenomenon can affect the penis as well, but it can in no way be considered a consequence of aging, but rather of deleterious behavior. The penis must be kept active.

As we've observed in the previous chapters, what the various stages of life have in common is the importance of hygiene throughout the genital area. This is even more the case in an old man: indeed it triggers a virtuous cycle because it encourages the full correspondence of the body which in turn encourages this care. Unfortunately, however, the opposite path has gained ground: hygiene is neglected, leading to certain penile dysfunctions or pathologies, which consequently cause pain or erectile difficulties, and through a domino effect people definitively cease taking care of their penis, giving it up for dead. This facilitates its exposure to infections, such as balanitis: this, if neglected, can degenerate into phimosis.

Our general state of health is quite influential. For example, in the presence of motor handicaps—not necessarily connected to the passage of time—it can be difficult to take proper care of one's genital hygiene, and thus infections risk becoming more frequent. It's crucial to be sure that someone sees to the health of our penis, sliding back the foreskin daily to wash and prevent the depositing of bacteria.

For a bed-ridden senior the doctor usually prefers the use of the **catheter** to the adult diaper. It's a silicone tube that's inserted along the urethra to connect directly into the bladder and is a great ally against incontinence. My answer to the question is that it's always better to incline toward the catheter, taking care to replace it every 20–30 days. If kept clean, the catheter creates far fewer complications than a diaper which, despite today being far more practical and anallergenic than in the past, nevertheless requires being changed multiple times a day, increasing the risk of infection.

If the body is healthy, fit and in good shape, the penis, too, remains in excellent condition. Vice versa, in two men of the same age, a man who is still sexually active has a greater life expectancy than one who has "hung up" his penis.

Let's not forget that our tool is the barometer of our health: a correct lifestyle is a key factor in prevention. A person in this age range must—I say it peremptorily—practice regular physical exercise, without exaggerating but getting out of the house and avoid a sedentary lifestyle. If a man who's no spring chicken is in shape and has good mobility, it's correct him to practice some sporting activity. Obviously it will be a good idea to choose "mild" sports, such as swimming, gym exercises (preferably with a trainer's supervision), outdoor walking and, why not, dancing. Vice versa, soccer or cycling are dangerous sports due to the potential for trauma—including of the pelvic region.

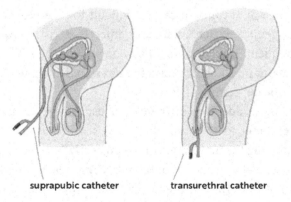

suprapubic catheter   transurethral catheter

Figure n. 25—Suprapubic and Transurethral Catheter

For individuals who are healthy and able to perform motor activities, certain exercises to **reinforce the pelvic floor** can be useful for keeping the penis, intestine and bladder in shape and under control.

The area concerned extends from the pubis to the coccyx and that muscles that compose it support both the bladder and the terminal part of the rectum. They can be weakened by a plurality of factors, from simple aging to the after-effects of an operation—typically of the prostate—from heavy labor to obesity, even a chronic cough. In order to really strengthen them, the specific exercises must be done with regularity, every day and for a sufficiently long period of time—at least four–six months.

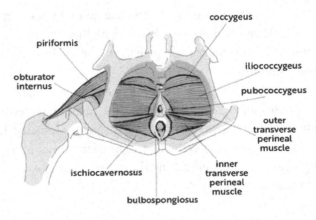

Figure n. 26— Muscles of the Pelvic Floor

Now imagine me in the shoes of a personal trainer, or an aqua gym instructor if you prefer, while I dictate the rhythm for performing your exercises. The suggested program calls for various series of voluntary contractions of the muscles, alternated with pauses of relaxation, with repetitions of a minimum of ten times. Ideally the training sessions should be repeated multiple times a day, in order to prevent, or at least, fight, the unpleasant problem of **incontinence**, often originating in prostate problems.

You should then pay attention to the proper cadence in the rhythms of waking and sleep, because rest, too, balanced in quality and quantity, takes on great importance.

Sleeping is crucial for our well-being, at any age. It's a need that diminishes with age, but our organism needs to be able to count on a set a of continuative rest—without, for instance, the discomfort of having to get up continually to go to the bathroom to urinate.

For an elderly man, six hours of continuous sleep would be an optimal rest interval.

Unfortunately, a man with prostate pathologies can find himself waking up in the middle of the night as many as five or six times, and this makes the quality, as well as the quantity, of his sleep plummet.

Lack of rest also has a further side effect. The reduction of REM phases also reduces the space for involuntary erection, that natural exercise so important for the penis's tonicity. This is one of the reasons why at the first signs of nocturia, of the irritating stimulus to get up during the night to urinate, a urological consult is necessary.

Tearing Down Prejudices

Antonio is sixty-seven years old and for some time has been waking up frequently at night to urinate. He began getting up two or three times a night, but recently it's increased to as many as five or six.

This prevents him from getting an extended period of rest,

and consequently he's rarely able to get up early to water his vege-table garden, before the summer sun gets too hot.

He decides to deal with the situation, but he has a problem. His trusted doctor is on vacation and in his place is a female substi-tute from outside the city. He found out from Luigi, who went to pick up his high-blood-pressure medication prescriptions and high-tailed it out of there.

Antonio swears to himself that he won't step foot in the clinic before Dr. Franzucchi's return. His friend's warning saved him from what he would have perceived as an embarrassing situation and, even more importantly, from relying on a women for prob-lems that concern his penis, of which she certainly knew very little.

But things become untenable when the need to use the bath-room so frequently makes him miss not one but two goals during his favorite team's match, while his friends celebrate at the sports bar's tables. The only short-term solution that he can think of is to ask for advice from Fabio, son of an acquaintance of his and his trusted pharmacist. Fabio, who knows what he's talking about and is aware of Antonio's limits, suggests he have a urological examination as soon as possible, because his condition requires further tests.

Fabio writes him the number of my office on a piece of paper and he calls to set an appointment. On the scheduled day he comes in. Naturally he hasn't told his wife.

"Hello, doctor, you were recommended to me by a mutual friend, Fab—" he falls silent mid-phrase and freezes in the doorway.

"Hello, Antonio. Please come in, make yourself comfortable."

"Oh, sorry, they didn't tell me we had company," he holds the door open for my colleague, seated next to me.

"No, not to worry, Sabrina is a resident in the Faculty of Urology and she'll be conducting the examination with me. You were talking about Fabio, sure, he's a dear patient of mine. So what brings you here?" Antonio doesn't answer and I struggle to understand what's going on. After a few moments he gets his courage up and resumes speaking.

"For a while now I've been waking up during the night because I feel the need to pee frequently and a sort of burning in my . . . sorry, can she step outside?"

Now I understand: the problem is Sabrina, the fact that she's a woman. I calmly explain to Antonio that I certainly could send the resident out, but this wouldn't be in anyone's interest. Not hers, since she'd miss out on a learning opportunity, nor his, since he'd lose that of a double consult and doubly-thorough check-up of his prostate.

"Antonio, put your mind at ease. In fact, consider yourself lucky: two urologists for the price of one!"

The patients gradually gives in, but from this moment on he doesn't utter a word. In silence we proceed with the rectal examination. Sabrina gives me precise indications on the state of his prostate, which permit the clear diagnosis of prostatitis, caught in time to be treated.

56% of the students in the Faculty of Medicine are female, a number that's destined to grow in time. One of the fields in which women struggle to establish themselves is urology, and the reason is to be sought in the still-widespread taboos, especially among more elderly patients.

What's always important to remember is that a doctor is a doctor, and when they are exercising their profession they area sexless. Residents in particular need to learn the tools of the trade and, to do so, need to observe in the field, without being hindered, Why aren't men in the world of gynecology looked at with the same mistrust?

The nutritional aspect is strategic. We Italians have the

advantage of being accustomed to the Mediterranean diet, but we need to pay attention not to overdo it with carbohydrates. It's good to vary the menu, eating a bit of everything, and keeping in mind that calorie consumption cannot be the same as that of a forty-year-old.

The contribution of water is important as well: you need to drink a lot. Water, that is, but a glass of red wine with meals, with its rich contribution of polyphenols, is still considered a panacea. It contrasts free radicals and prevents the oxidation at the foundation of phenomena of arteriosclerotic degeneration.

Lastly, it's important not to forget that the penis is directly affected by alterations in levels of glycemia, cholesterol and triglycerides. If our values aren't in the norm, we might notice this precisely from imperfections in penile functionality. To maintain a healthy prostate, certain vegetables are recommended, those we usually avoid cooking because they're smellier than others, such as broccoli, cauliflower and cabbage, which contain sulforaphane, an ally of the prostate gland.

If up to now we have talked about the general functioning of the penis, I'd now like to focus on the sexual sphere. Indeed it's still too common to think that, past a certain age, the penis becomes a useless appendage.

If an individual is healthy and doesn't take any drugs with side effects on the sexual sphere, his performance will remain unaltered. Should he, on the other hand, suffer from any pathology—hypertension, diabetes, Parkinson's, endocrine or cardiovascular diseases—the penis's functionality could be affected. From my standpoint, caring for a patient of seventy-five or older poses fewer problems than for someone in their fifties. In the elderly man, indeed, the problem, paradoxically, are simpler, even basic, while in an middle-aged man a given symptom could conceal a whole series of potentially serious situations, which need to be analyzed and discarded one by one.

At the beginning of the chapter we mentioned how much the term "andropause" is used in the media despite being devoid of scientific foundation. It's often confused with the question linked to the production of testosterone. This a fundamental hormone for male sexuality: among its purposes, beside the control of insulin-resistance (strategic for protecting the organism from diabetes), fighting depression, protecting against osteoporosis and vascular problems, there lies in fact the regulation of sexual desire. In the man, testosterone is generated in the gonads (testicles), by Leydig cells and, although in lesser quantity, by the suprarenal cortex.

Around age fifty, the male organism's standard levels naturally begin to fall. If the descent stops within a natural range we speak of **age-correlated hypogonadism**—a state also defined as *Late Onset Hypogonadism*: the debate on the possibility of intervening with a targeted therapy or leaving things as they are is still open. If the descent continues beyond the minimum level, on the other hand, it's a case of **simple hypogonadism**, a pathological situation that we'll look into further in a dedicated section.

A cause of the fall in testosterone can be **metabolic syndrome**, also known as **insulin-resistance syndrome.** This is a clinical condition associated with a high risk of cardio-circulatory pathologies and it's characterized by a concurrence of multiple factors, including arterial hypertension, high rates of glycemia and triglycerides in the blood, a low level of HDL cholesterol (high-density lipoproteins—"good" cholesterol), an abdominal circumference greater than 102 cm. In individuals with glycemia and triglyceride values in the norm, testosterone is released into the blood circulation through the metabolism; in those affected by metabolic syndrome, on the other hand, this is "captured" by the excess fat, thus remaining unutilized, with connected problems including the increase of erectile dysfunctions.

But that's not the end of it. Beyond the **endocrine system**, the **cardio-circulatory system** must be kept under close surveillance as well. The penis's vascularization is articulated in arteries and veins, on the surface as well as deeper in, from which branch off increasingly thin vessels. An obstructed blood vessel in the penis can cause problems in the sexual sphere, typically on the order of erectile dysfunction, and thus sound an alarm to which it would be wise to pay attention: the closure of that little vessel could be the prelude to a phenomenon that will appear in a few years in the coronary arteries.

An episode of erectile dysfunction should not be repressed because it could save us from a future heart attack. This indication is naturally valid at any age, but even more so from sixty on. This doesn't mean, however, that we should start panicking the first time we "misfire."

PATHOLOGIES

In old age, urological pathologies are on average more common than for adolescent and adult males. For three main reasons: due to **neglected medical conditions**, which after years swiftly decline; to **chronic diseases** of other body systems with consequences on the genital organ; and to a **natural wear** caused by time and to which the penis isn't immune.

Most of the pathologies, however, are not the exclusive consequence of time's passing but of the individual's conscious behavior over the course of his life. And not just in terms of diet and lifestyle. I'm thinking, for example, of a man who has never had regular examinations and checkups and who, like a bolt from the blue, discovers he's suffering from something now at an advanced stage.

Prevention and information are the most powerful weapons at our disposal: one of the clearest indicators of this statement is the number of elderly patients who contract STDs in old age. People often think, "Well, if I haven't gotten anything until now it means I'm immune, nothing will happen to me," but an elderly penis is less reactive, and thus more subject to micro-traumas and diseases.

The data confirm it. The frequency of HIV is growing particularly among patients over sixty, less sensitive to using condoms than younger people. Prevention through protection is thus always valid, partly because it's the only weapon effective against STDs.

It should be said that the elderly man, more than his younger counterpart, suffers in the use of the condom. It's more difficult for an imperfectly-erect penis to wear a condom. But there's a solution for this as well. There are drugs that aid both the erection and the consequent use of the condom. Let's always protect ourselves and our partner, even when we have white hair and a denture.

Now we'll take a broad look at the **most frequent pathologies** of the penis in elderhood and the symptoms that characterize them.

Balanitis

Typically due to **scarce personal hygiene or unprotected sexual activity.**

Cleansers, creams, or doctor-prescribed are capable of combatting it.

Paraphimosis

As in the child and adolescent, the foreskin is unable to its normal position covering the glans.

For the elderly, the cause is linked to **bad personal hygiene**, a **previous balanitis** or the **loss of tissue elasticity**. It can be resolved through a manual maneuver or, in the most difficult cases, with a simple operation.

Orchiepididymitis

It appears with an intense and sudden pain in the testicle, caused by infection or inflammation.

Treatment is exclusively by antibiotics, administered orally. In the elderly man it often leads to a **reactive hydrocele**, at which point the solution is surgical.

Hypogonadism

The diagnosis of hypogonadism includes the analysis of the symptoms and lab tests that confirm the **deficiency of testosterone**. Among the most common symptoms: the reduction of libido and erectile dysfunction; the thinning out of body hair and the slowing down of beard regrowth; the increase of weight, visceral fat and waist circumference; the reduction of sebaceous secretion and a certain cutaneous dryness; gynecomastia; osteoporosis.

Several studies have demonstrated that testosterone concentrations diminish gradually with age.

Hypogonadism affects 4.2% between 30 and 50 and 8.4% between 50 and 79. Nevertheless, the terminology to explain the relation with aging is controversial. At present we prefer to speak of **Late-Onset Hypogonadism**, or **LOH.** According to recent data, the presence of LOH in males over 70 seems to be at least 20%.

The open question in the scientific field is focused on whether and how to intervene in the presence of this pathology, which is at least in part natural, evaluating the benefits of treatment with testosterone and the risks associated with such an intervention.

A replacement therapy for testosterone should be undertaken only when there is a confirmed diagnosis of severe hypogonadism—at the testicular level—based in turn on below-norm testosterone levels and a simultaneous validation from clinical tests. No treatment ought to be initiated, on the other hand, with testosterone level within the norm, even in the presence of symptoms correlated with hypogonadism. This is because the administration of testosterone leads to significant side effects, including making the blood less fluid, with connected significant risks of developing cardio-circulatory pathologies, including strokes. Among other things, pharmacological testosterone cannot be taken orally, but necessitates injections.

Only recently have latest-generation products in the form of gels appeared on the market.

Applied with the frequency suggested by the patient's clinical profile, they make it possible to keep testosterone within levels considered normal. Nevertheless, at the current state of knowledge and available therapies, the guiding principle remains that of caution. Testosterone should not be prescribed automatically to every individual who displays a deficiency: I insist on the fact that the side effects can be quite serious.

Personally, I prefer to begin by suggesting a program of

physical exercise or nice walks, because a healthy and balanced lifestyle really does help a lot. In any case, considering as well the limits of the data available to us, I underline that any pharmacological therapy must be initiated only at the end of a targeted diagnostic procedure and under a specialist's close supervision.

Incontinence

This condition is statistically quite widespread, particularly among men who suffer from an **enlarged prostate.** The latter, in fact, when it increases in volume, can slow down or even block the passage of urine, causing at a later moment the sudden need to urinate. The stimulus can be so intense that it doesn't always give you enough time to reach a toilet. Incontinence almost seems to close the circle of our life, bringing us back to when, as little boys, we had yet to recognize the stimulus to pee. But this doesn't justify the indiscriminate recourse to the adult diaper, other roads should be tried beforehand.

Some diseases typical of the elderly man, such as Parkinson's, include incontinence among their symptoms. Nevertheless, it can have different causes: a prostate operation, or better, a radical prostatectomy (which is now undertaken up to age 75) to treat prostate cancer, or a pelvic trauma with conse- quent damage to the urethral sphincter. In this case we speak of **stress incontinence** and the classic example is that of small and involuntary losses of urine after a sneeze or cough. In these cases we can intervene surgically, positioning a contoured bandage to replace the urethra's supporting musculature that's been compromised.

Then there's **urge incontinence**, which is the most common form and occurs when the bladder contracts at the wrong time, giving the sensation of needing to urinate immediately. This stimulus can also be deceptive, especially if we've just emptied our bladder. This is resolved through an operation on the prostate, main culprit for this problem.

Overflow incontinence, on the other hand, concerns urine losses that occur when the bladder is unable to empty properly. It's usually caused by an enlarged prostate or urethral shrinkage. If neglected, it can lead to an emergency widespread among elderly patients, acute urinary retention, which we'll look at in the section dedicated to emergencies.

Lastly there is **total incontinence**, or the continuous loss of urine due to complete deficiency of the sphincter, often linked to neurological ailments.

For all these cases we have seen that there are treatments, which vary according to the incontinence we experience and the organs involved. Today there are many options to resolve the problem. Before surrendering to the adult diaper or catheter it's important to seek out the most appropriate solution. In the most serious cases you can make recourse to an artificial sphincter, in which a ring is positioned around the urethra that permits you to regain continence. It's still little talked-about, considered to be a niche surgical option, but it's necessary to know it exists. For slight cases of incontinence it's important, on the other hand, to train the pelvic floor, as we saw in the "Upkeep" section.

Prostate Pathologies

In this period the most common pathologies are undoubtedly those that concern the **prostate.**

It's only right and proper, therefore, to recall its anatomy and how it works.

The prostate's key function is containing the prostatic liquid, which composes 90% of the seminal fluid released with ejaculation—that's right, contrary to popular belief, the ejaculate doesn't come directly from the testicles but rather from here—and protects on the one hand the genital apparatus as a whole, on the other the spermatozoa in particular. The liquid, in fact, is composed of valuable substances: proteins, lipids, prostaglandins, hormones, fructose, Vitamin C, carnitine, zinc and others still, useful for creating the perfect environment for the spermatozoon's survival.

It is, in short, a gland of the male body positioned just below the bladder and traversed by a section of the urethra. If an individual has problems with this gland, one of the first symptoms will be precisely that of difficulties urinating. The medical term is **dysuria,** or irritation linked to miction.

There are fundamentally three pathologies that can affect this gland: **prostatitis** (inflammation of the prostate), benign prostatic hypertrophy (the prostate grows, causing pressure on the urethra and making it more difficult for urine to come out) and **prostate cancer** (degeneration linked to the appearance of neoplastic cells).

The real problem is that they can also arise simultaneously. Clinical data indicate that, past the age of seventy-five, the concomitant presence of prostatitis and **benign prostatic hypertrophy** is extremely frequent. It should be observed, however, that while for the latter there is a link of a familiar (genetic) nature, the same is not true for prostatitis.

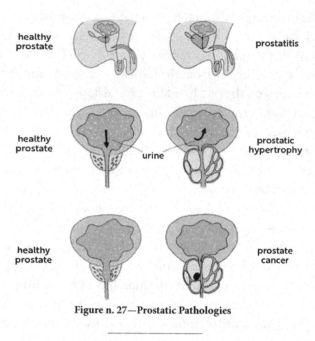

Figure n. 27—Prostatic Pathologies

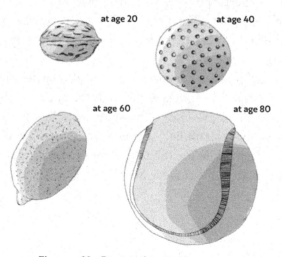

Figure n. 28—Prostate size at various ages

As men age, the risk of developing prostate cancer is very high: between seventy-five and eighty it's roughly 50%. The European Association of Urology's guidelines say that, over the age of 75, it no longer makes sense to look for it, it's probably there. It is almost always, however, a carcinoma with a very slow evolution, capable of developing clinical problems only 10–20 years after its appearance, when the end of the life cycle, in any case, has already been reached. The pathology's particularly elevated rate, nevertheless, mustn't scare us. In fact it explains why it's considered a quasinatural situation.

Frequency differs according to ethnic groups: Blacks have a greater predisposition than whites. Moreover, when a population changes continents it acquires the percentage of risk of the communities already residing in the new territory. Social, cultural and environmental input such as diet, lifestyle and pollution levels have a great deal of influence. Then there's the hereditary factor to consider, to the extent that if a patient has a father or brother affected by the pathology it's a good idea for him to undergo periodic, targeted check-ups.

The **symptoms** of the three pathologies are similar. That of prostatitis is dysuria, or difficulty urinating, accompanied by burning during miction and a scattered pain in the perineum, testicles and suprapubic region.

That of prostatic hypertrophy is nocturia. You have to get up multiple times a night to go to the bathroom, but when you get there the urine doesn't come out immediately, you have to wait a few seconds. The stream also presents characteristics of "hypovalidity": it's weak and points decidedly downward (reason for which my patients often tell me, "I do it on my slippers"). A further symptom can be, contrarily, incontinence. In terms of blood tests, the alteration of PSA values can indicate the presence of an ongoing prostatic hypertrophy.

Prostate cancer, on the other hand, is **asymptomatic** and for this reason more devious. Only in advances stages do you notice symptoms linked to metastases that affect the bones, and thus a very acute and uncontrolled pain, rare situation in part because great progress has been made in prevention and early diagnosis. In this sense, as for all asymptomatic pathologies, constant monitoring takes on great importance, particularly through the PSA test, starting from age 50 (and 45 in the presence of prostate cancer cases in the family). It's useful to remember that we mustn't be unjustifiably afraid: screening doesn't create the disease, it identifies it, if it exists, and the sooner we do it, the better. Let's also remember here that the PSA is not a univocal indicator of the tumor's presence and thus it's necessary to investigate an abnormal value further with your urologist.

In any case the diagnosis occurs in very simple manner. First comes anamnesis, or the analysis of the patient's history, followed in the clinic by a rectal exploration to verify prostate size. In normal conditions it should be the size of a chestnut, while in the presence of a benign prostatic hypertrophy it becomes more similar to a tangerine, taking on the size of an orange in very advanced cases. If there's a prostatitis, the urologist's finger perceives an anomalous warmth; in the case of a tumor, finally, it feels the presence of a nodule.

Normally, to facilitate the rectal exploration, the patient is asked to lie down on his side. The urologist, with a well-lubricated glove, inserts a finger in the rectum and examines the prostate as a whole (the median lobe and the two lateral lobes), to evaluate its flexibility and size. The operation shouldn't cause pain (I say this to put all you worried folks' minds at ease).

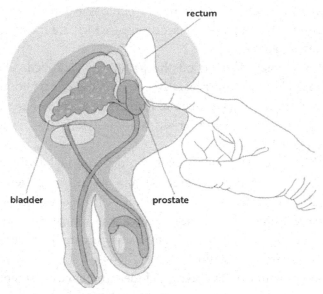

Figure n. 29— Prostate exam

I, on the other hand, examine the patient on his feet, having him bend over. The reason is simple: in this position the prostate is closer to my finger and the diagnosis more precise. In my experience, for the patient it's less psychologically affecting to lie down, since the clinic bed immediately puts him in the condition of someone with an issue and thus makes more inclined to be examined; but it isn't always a winning choice. The examination only lasts a few seconds, and pre-exploration anxiety and fears vanish immediately.

To be certain of the presence of a prostatic tumor it is later necessary to undergo a biopsy, or a tissue sampling. First, however, the patient has a multiparametric MRI. The biopsy is carried out with local anesthesia, at a clinic or as outpatient care at a hospital, and lasts just a few minutes.

An ultrasound probe is inserted into the rectum to take several tissue samples—at least twelve—which are then sent to the lab for analysis.

The therapy depends on the pathology identified. In the 75-year-old man with **prostatitis,** it is first necessary to identify the trigger. If it's a bacterial form, the patient is started on antibiotics. If it's an abacterial form, lifestyle factors must be investigated.

The suggested protocol calls for drinking a lot of water, getting regular physical exercise and following a diet that focuses on specific foods and beverages. It becomes necessary to avoid white wine and beer, pepper and hot pepper (which contains capsaicin, use for the circulatory system but harmful if you suffer from prostatitis).

Some claim that it's also a good idea to reduce consumption of cured meats and coffee, or adopt a rigid diet, though scientific evidence for this is lacking. In my view, common sense and proportion need to prevail.

A good diet, as we've seen, should be sufficient for the requirements of minerals, vitamins and proteins that our genital system needs to function correctly.

It's also true that increasingly often we see commercials that push us to consider assistance; for prostatitis we could use several nutritional and phytotherapeutic supplements such as those containing *Boswellia* (an anti-inflammatory and analgesic), *Serenoa Repens* (which improves the prostate gland's functioning and stimulates the urinary flow), zinc (which helps the quality and mobility of the spermatozoa and diminishes the risk of cancer), Vitamin D (which helps keep the cells healthy) and selenium (which facilitates spermatogenesis).

The debate is still open on these supplements. The main problem is that the data we have are incomplete and don't provide a sufficient perspective to draw conclusions. To establish whether a preparation benefits the prostate or not today we still look to a study—a bit dated now—called MTOPS. Its value stems from the breadth of the sample and the duration of the measurements (over four and a half years).

The MTOPS highlighted that the drugs in question begin to produce effects only after at least a year from the first use, and that therefore a new drug should be tested for a minimum period of one or two years before being put on the market. This can require significant investments often beyond the range of the supplement companies. Experiments were thus done on the supplements for three-six months, too short a period of time. Does this mean that supplements are good? Or bad? Or that they might have no effect? In the worst hypothesis they do nothing, they're certainly not harmful. Personally, I use them and recommend them.

The widespread use of supplements underlines a greater awareness of the pathology, which is positive. A broader consciousness of this issue even outside the scientific community could be an opportunity to explore the territory more thoroughly and drive pharmaceutical companies to conduct longer experiments.

We now move to the **therapy for benign prostatic hypertrophy.** It includes particularly the use of:

- **Alpha blockers.** Used when the symptoms concern difficulty in emptying the bladder, because they produce a relaxation of the bladder neck's musculature, improving the urine flow. The side effects, however, include retrograde ejaculation.
- **5-ARIs (5-alpha reductase inhibitors).** Used in patients over age 75. Finasteride and dutasteride (two 5-ARIs) inhibit the growth of the prostatic adenoma

and can even reduce its volume by 20%. Side effects include a fall in libido, erectile dysfunction and the disappearance of ejaculation, but these appear only in 10% of cases—even if, due to the so-called "nocebo" effect, if you read the instructions carefully you have the perception of feeling at least one of them, given that they are very delicate effects and susceptible to psychological conditioning.

- **Antimuscarinics.** Used in cases of bladder over-activity and thus incontinence stemming from prostatic hypertrophy. They aren't prescribed if the patient isn't able to empty his bladder completely. They can be used together with alpha blockers.
- **Phytotherapics and nutraceutics.** These are the same supplements we introduced in the treatment of prostatitis, whose advantage is there lack of repercussions on the sexual sphere.
- **Phosphodiesterase-5 inhibitors** (PDE-5). One of the most common in treating prostatic hypertrophy is Tadalafil, which, among other things, relaxes the pelvic floor, easing pressure on the prostate. It has been proven to improve symptoms of dysuria, even if it's used principally in treating erectile dysfunction. As they say, two birds with one stone.

If these treatments don't work or the side effects are greater than their benefits, regaining correct bladder functioning can be achieved through several techniques of micro-surgery. These are endoscopic operations that use the opening of the penis, reach the urethra at the prostate and proceed to broaden the urinary duct.

Simplifying, we could compare the operation to the

widening of a tunnel that had partially narrowed. For example, the **TURP** (Transurethral Resection of the Prostate) is one of these, and lasts roughly one hour. In three or four days, the patient is sent home. For patients with significant blood clotting problems there are also micro-invasive techniques, including laser surgery.

GreenLight, to name one—whose name, among other things, resembles that of a superhero, as a patient of mine mentioned—reduces bleeding by healing up immediately and permitting release from the hospital the day after the operation. In this case as well, the passage offered by the urethra is exploited.

TURP and laser surgery preserve ejaculation, but they make it retrograde. Orgasm no longer leads to the release of sperm, which goes into the bladder. As far as pleasure goes nothing changes, but the patient can suffer evident psychological and fertility problems. In preparing the patient for the operation, therefore, it's correct to clarify these aspects, which might otherwise lead to frustration and discomfort in the post-op phase.

Thoroughly discuss all the possibilities with your doctor before the operation, to understand what the risks are and evaluate their relationship with the benefits. One more question is always better than one less.

In recent years there have appeared innovative technologies indicated for patients whose sexuality is still fully active. One technology that's the latest fashion is **Rezum**, which seems like GreenLight's evil adversary but is actually a device that uses water vapor to obtain the reduction of the prostatic lobes. To explain in greater detail, a micro-needle is used on the penis in order to create an entryway, moving backup before creating little perforations on the prostatic lobes. Water is then vaporized, taking care to position a catheter to be maintained for seven days. In a few weeks, the thermal effect generates a consistent reduction in prostatic volume and then a widening of the urethra. The entire operation requires just a few minutes, and the patient is released after a few hours.

The technology is certainly recommended for younger patients, but at the same time it permits the operation for patients over 90 with a permanent catheter, for whom a classic operation isn't recommended. To close the circle of superheroes and futuristic devices, recently even a robot has been developed—the **Aquabeam**—capable of removing the prostate in less than five minutes thanks to a stream of water shot at the speed of sound. In this case, too, ejaculation is preserved. Summing up, if you choose the classic endoscopic TURP, in 90% of cases it leads to retrograde ejaculation, due to which the semen no longer leaves the penis during ejaculation but ends up in the bladder. The consequence, then, is sterility, with a small chance of recovery. If you use the GreenLight laser, the chances for maintaining ejaculation increase significantly compared to the traditional operation. With the vaporization of the prostate via Rezum, ejaculation is preserved for nine patients out of ten, a percentage which increases slightly with the use of Aquabeam.

In hypertrophy operations the vascular nervous structures aren't touched, so erection is preserved. Only a small percentage of patients report problems of this type, which, however, aren't connected to the operation but to the aging process.

The therapy for prostate cancer is evaluated on the basis of various factors: the most important of them is certainly age, but also the tumor's degree of aggressiveness. Each case is unique and every man has his anamnesis, his history, his priorities, his expectations.

If the tumor is localized within the prostate, there are three possible ways forward:

1. **Watchful waiting.** Only for certain select cases, often those in which the biopsy only showed as tumoral one of the twelve or more samples taken, it's possible to implement a vigilant waiting period, during which periodic check-ups monitor the tumor's evolution or stabilization.
2. **Surgery.** The removal of the entire prostate gland and of the lymph nodes of the region (radical prostatectomy) is considered a curative operation. It can be carried out with a classic, open-air operation, with laparoscopy (using, that is, small perforations of the abdomen as the entrance channel) or even with robotic surgery, in the scope of which the instruments are moved via robot.
3. **Radiation therapy.** In low-risk tumors the results of the prostatectomy are comparable to those of radiation therapy, of which various typologies exist.

Unlike what happens elsewhere, when the prostatic tumor is in a metastatic state, hormonal therapy is preferred to chemotherapy. This, in fact, reduces the level of testosterone—the male hormone that stimulates the growth of the prostate tumor's cells—but brings with it side effects such as the fall or disappearance of sexual desire, impotence, hot flashes, weight increase, osteoporosis, the loss of muscle mass, and fatigue.

As we've observed, there isn't one of the three options that can be declared as the best, but in the case of a man over 75 radiation therapy is the first choice. Both the therapy and the monitoring share the adjective "active" to underline that nothing is left to chance and that it's important not to surrender passively to the disease's evolution without medical support.

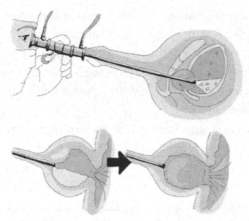

Figure n. 30—Prostate operation

Thanks to progress in robotization we can achieve far more satisfying results than those of a few years ago, in terms of both precision and effectiveness. But the treatment's future is connected more to radiation therapy than to surgery. The same progress, in fact, has benefitted the latter as well, which is more targeted and better controlled.

When the tumor is very aggressive, it's necessary to combine various therapies according to the profile and specificities of the patient (surgery, radiation therapy, hormonal therapy, chemotherapy, etc.) to block the tumor's development. We must never forget sexuality, which even in the case of a tumoral diagnosis must never be given up for dead. Being sexually active can help maintain a certain well-being and higher morale even during the therapy. More and more specialists are becoming conscious of this.

I want to clarify another aspect as well. The more "classic" prostate operations sacrifice ejaculation and provoke sterility. The operation calls for the removal of the elements in which the body produces spermatozoa, and this consequence is thus inevitable.

Well, this is a topic to evaluate with great care. Radiation therapy has consequences on the erectile mechanism and often leads to the development of hemorrhoids linked to a burning sensation. With the elimination of the prostate, we inevitably corrode the vascular mechanism, which can lead to problems not just in ejaculation but in erection as well and thus in sexual life as a whole.

The 3D and digital imaging technologies now available for microsurgery enable a view once unthinkable and contribute to reducing the risks associated with the operation. The percentage of preservation of erection—keeping in mind concurrent pathologies (diabetes, hypertension, etc.)—ranges today between 50 and 70% of cases.

In 2013 Dr. Riccardo Bartoletti and I carried out on a young patient the first-ever operation of laparoscopic surgery, with removal of the prostate and, simultaneously, placement of a penile implant. The basic line of reasoning is the same as the reconstruction of the breast following breast cancer. 8 years later, he and the other patients that have followed him have been able to return to a normal sexuality in as little as 3–4 weeks and their penis has remained its preoperation size, to the satisfaction of those concerned and their partners.

This type of operation is still not very common due to the high immediate costs and the reluctance of some colleagues linked to the risk of infection of the prosthesis, which, however, in the operation with Dr. Bartoletti, we completely belied.

The recovery time following an operation must naturally be considered, necessary before thinking about the solution of other derivative problems. For benign prostatic hypertrophy it's a matter of roughly 30 days; for prostate cancer up to 18 months of rest can be necessary. In my clinical experience, within six months it's possible to establish the best treatment for resolving the potential erectile dysfunction issues induced.

Whatever therapy is used, I suggest beginning immediately a sort of "penis rehabilitation," because if it stays inactive for too long it tends to develop forms of internal fibrosis that will undermine its functionality. The mere inactivity, and consequent fibrosis, could lead to a shortening of several centimeters

The best exercise for the penis is obviously erection. Rehabilitation consists, therefore, in this: seeking opportunities that induce the mechanism. Whether it's sex or masturbation is secondary: the important thing, in these conditions, is the exercise in itself.

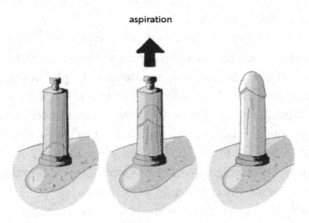

aspiration

Figure n. 31—Penis Pump

Just like in CrossFit, there are specific devices for training your erection as well. A tool that's easy to use is the **vacuum device:** by exploiting the vacuum created by a suction pump, it makes the erection occur mechanically. The device consists of a large silicone cylinder inside of which you place the flaccid penis. Via a manual or electric pump a negative pressure of 100–150 mmHg is created that causes blood to flow to the penis, it's like applying a section cup to your skin, you'll see right away with the naked eye that the area becomes deep red, testifying to the influx of blood.

Erectile Dysfunction

We've already investigated the question of erectile dysfunction in the adult male, but we also naturally find it later in the aging process. A pharmacological therapy can provide erectile support after an operation on the genital area. It's important to know, in fact, that drugs for postop erectile dysfunction are provided by the National Health Service. Tuscany was the first region to enact this absolutely necessary proposal, which was later extended to the entire national territory.

All the drugs belonging to the family of PDE-5 inhibitors—those, therefore, that descend from Viagra and include Cialis, Levitra and Spedra—are safe in old age as well (for more on this topic, see the previous chapter). These are substantially enzymes that, in the presence of a sexual stimulus—visual, olfactory, or tactile—are activated and influence the smooth musculature of the penis, which relaxes. In this way, by increasing the flow of blood in the existing cavities of the cavernous tissue, they facilitate the erectile mechanism via vasodilation.

The process isn't influenced by age and presents no drawbacks. Obviously individuals with circulatory problems should conduct a thorough evaluation of them with their doctor. An individual with cardiac pathologies, for example, could be at risk less for the effect of the drugs than because sexual activity—especially when intense—represents physical strain in itself. Viagra, and with it the other drugs of the same family, doesn't induce any dangerous side effects, but rather encourages people to make love, but if they aren't able to sustain this activity then, yes, the patient can encounter serious consequences.

The right path, then, must start from a heart check-up. If the result confirms that its state of health is good and that there are no significant dangers connected to potential physical strain, then all clear to use these drugs.

At present there are only two known contraindications to the use of PDE-5 inhibitors: the simultaneous use with nitrates, for the treatment of various cardio-circulatory pathologies via patch or sublingually, intravenously, or rectally, and the presence of retinitis pigmentosa, an eye ailment which Viagra can causa to degenerate. Patients who suffer from it are clearly aware of this aspect. Nevertheless I suggest never relying on self-prescription or using Viagra as an aphrodisiac or "fun pill," but always to turn to a doctor for the prescription, following a prompt visit.

In the chapter dedicated to adulthood we observed that to contrast erectile dysfunction it's also possible to make recourse to localized injections on the penis. This solution has a high rate of abandonment, since it's often painful. As a last choice, if you're looking for a definitive and permanent solution, I recommend an implant, at any age. The operation consists of placing inside the penile shaft a hydraulic system composed of two cylinders that artificially reproduce the corpora cavernosa.

It's simple, takes roughly an hour, and can be done either in outpatient care or with overnight hospitalization. The only risk is that of infection, found, furthermore, only in 2% of cases. If you use a simple prosthesis—one-piece—the consistency of the two corpora cavernosa is constant, thus sufficiently rigid to support penetration but at the same time flexible enough to be managed in daily life. When two- or three-piece, or hydraulic, implants are used, the control device, a little pump, is placed inside the scrotum, and the liquid reservoir in the abdomen. A closed-circuit system is created that permits the penis's erection when the liquid is transferred inside the two cylinders;

vice versa, there's a return to the flaccid state when the liquid is poured back into the reservoir.

Thanks to these systems, four weeks after the operation you can resume a satisfying sexual activity.

The insertion of the implant doesn't cause pain, except for the immediate surgical follow-up, common to any other operation and manageable pharmacologically.

The only complication can be due to a malfunction of the prosthesis, due to which a surgical revision could be necessary.

But this is very rare.

Unacceptable Behavior

The protagonist of this story is named Oreste. He's thirty-nine years old, so he can't be considered an elderly man. Yet it's important to look at his story here to underline how incorrect behavior and a neglected pathology can degenerate and alter someone's quality of life for good. In his case, not just carelessly but with intent. When he comes to see me he's very tense, his hands are shaking and he's visibly sweating. I sense his profound terror for my entire professional category long before he's able to confess it to me. But what strikes me most is that he tends to normalize his behavior.

"Coming here scares everybody, doesn't it? Plus it's my first time."

He even asks me for time to get used to the idea of pulling his pants and underwear down, in a sort of mystic meditation. Talking about what the problem is, naturally, is out of the question. "See for yourself, it'll be faster that way."

After a few jerks backward, I'm able to examine him. On his foreskin are small warts, the rooster crests, at an advanced stage and likely due to an HPV infection.

I prescribe a semen test to be sure of the diagnosis and set a simple electrocoagulation operation to remove the outgrowths.

A month later, Oreste emails me the result of the analyses that confirm a Human Papilloma Virus infection. I set an appointment to proceed with the operation, exhorting him to always use a condom and maintain this habit at least until he tests negative for the virus, a period that could vary from six months to two years.

But Oreste doesn't show up for his appointment and, given the situation, I call him personally and say that if he's just a few minutes late I can take the next patient and see him after. With a hesitant tone of voice he tells me that he's at work, that he forgot. So we set another appointment, but once again he fails to come in.

Despite my repeated insistence on the seriousness of the situation and the possibility of a degeneration in the near future, he repeats his actions not once, but five times in the space of a few months. A year has now passed and I've lost touch with him completely. My hope is that he's decided to turn to another specialist, someone who managed to ease his mind and act before he could go into hiding, and above all that he's informed any partners of the risk of contagion.

These are cases in which it saddens me not to be able to force people to come in. Irresponsibility towards oneself and others can have unimaginable consequences, far more serious than anyone's fear of doctors.

It's important never to postpone an examination or operation, but rather to act immediately, especially when the diagnosis is clear.

Penile Cancer

Let's dedicate a final section to **penile cancer,** a pathology now quite rare in Western countries and that develops in men with poor personal hygiene. An HPV (Human Papilloma Virus) infection is the principal risk factor. It often appears with small lesions on the penis and the diagnosis is made exclusively via biopsy.

Once it's confirmed, it's necessary to evaluate how far the disease has spread. If it's in an initial phase, operating with a laser can be sufficient. More serious cases, which are quite rare, can necessitate the partial or complete removal of the penis, followed by radiation therapy and chemotherapy.

Correct hygiene and the surgical removal of any condylomas linked to HPV are the only possible prevention steps. In all my years of medical experience I've encountered roughly thirty patients with penile cancer, but one of the most striking cases occurred one day during my shift at the ER.

I often tell the story, not just to exorcise that moment verging on the surreal, but also to emphasize yet again the need for daily penile care and hygiene.

EMERGENCIES

One of the most widespread emergencies of the male genital apparatus is **acute urinary retention,** or the impossibility to urinate. If the presence of phimosis isn't detected in the patient, the cause could lie in a urethral stenosis or a malfunction of the prostate.

The positioning of a vesical catheter excludes the question of stenosis and temporarily resolves the prostatic problem. However, if it concerns the urethra, an operation is required to position an **epicist**—a catheter in the bladder from the abdomen. Those with prostate problems often fear urinary retention, but this only happens if we check ourselves periodically.

If we notice we're drinking without feeling the stimulus to urinate, this should be an alarm bell. Among the other symptoms we can number burning, urine that struggles to come out, what we would call "a drop at a time," and in the most serious cases high fever as well, caused by the urine's return to the kidneys.

If, finally, we notice that an elderly man's diaper is always quite dry we should consider a consult with a urologist or family doctor. The ordinary upkeep of the prostate goes a long way to reducing the frequency of retention.

Hurry Up, It's Late

It's Friday evening, I've just arrived with my family at a hotel outside of town. The screen on my cellphone lights up as I'm in the elevator.

Franco, one of my patients, informs me with a worried tone that he's been struggling to urinate since this morning. He's 71 years old, and I've known him for 10. The last time, we conducted a rectal exploration that confirmed the need to proceed with a prostate operation for an onset of prostatic hypertrophy, which he promptly put off to some future date.

"Franco, listen to me, it's nothing serious, but have them take you to the ER. They'll give you a catheter, it's the only thing you can and must do to empty your bladder. Then I'll see you next week and we'll decide how to proceed."

"No, doctor. I only want you to examine me. If you have room we'll wait for Monday, otherwise I'll see you Tuesday."

"Monday is too late for your bladder. If you want I'll talk to a colleague on call and have you examined tomorrow morning."

"Don't bother, I only called to find out if it was normal, I'm not in pain, I was just concerned." Despite my inflexibility and insistence, I'm not able to convince him. I hang up with the promise to see him Monday.

I wake up early the next day and, as predicted, I find a message from Franco.

I'm at the ER, Doc. You were right. But don't tell my wife about this message: after forty years of marriage, she still thinks I'm incapable of saying it.

The majority of cases of urinary retention are due to an enlargement of the prostate which blocks the bladder's proper functioning. But this doesn't happen suddenly, it's a gradual process of which our body gives us increasingly insistent signals, mostly connected to miction. Patients often try to avoid the matter, hoping it will take care of itself, believing in the curative power of "Just wait a few more hours." Don't wait, don't postpone, don't deny the evidence.

It's important to have a urologist of reference, who knows your clinical history and can inform you of the changes underway in your genital system.

Rarer, on the other hand, are cases of **pharmacological priapism.** The term priapism means when the erect penis doesn't return to the state of flaccidity. It's first necessary to place ice on the pubis and avoid immobility. Better to move around, such as going up and down stairs to facilitate the blood flow.

If the problem doesn't resolve itself on its own within a few hours it's necessary to go to the ER for an urgent examination. From the anamnesis conducted on that occasion we'll be able to figure out what type of priapism it is. If it originates in a trauma—a fall or, as is often the case, banging against the crossbar of a bicycle—the problem can be resolved with selective embolization, which is merely the blockage of several blood vessels of the corpora cavernosa. If the cause is of the pharmacological sort or derives from blood diseases, the solution will require an immediate operation. The consequences of a priapism that isn't immediately resolved can be serious and damage the erectile mechanism.

A situation of extreme clinical alarm, connected to bad overall conditions, a serious genital infection or diabetes is **Fournier gangrene.** It's an extremely rare condition: to give you some idea, most urologists never encounter it in their entire professional career. It is a sepsis (putrefactive gangrene) of the genitals, which demands an immediate destructive operation. The most serious cases can lead to the removal of so much tissue that only the external envelope of the two testicles is left intact, in the hopes that the scrotum is reformed over time. If you don't operate immediately, the mortality rate is particularly high (roughly 40%). If the patient has already entered a septic state, the risk of death rises to 80%. The appropriate therapy is indicated on an individual basis at the conclusion of the specialist's examination.

We come to the end of this section. On the one hand we've gathered positive and encouraging signs: medicine has now drastically reduced the number of hopeless situations, and its progress continues. On the other, the image of the white-bearded grandfather with his grandchildren on his knees seems, truth be told, obsolete.

We might not realize it because the steps forward have occurred over time, but the last 20 years have brought us one success after another. Those who have benefitted most, clearly, are adult males, but so have elderly men. This doesn't mean that their role in daily life has changed: the people are the same as before, but they can now do more rather than having to settle for regrets. Ultimately, we are witnessing a process of enrichment of society as a whole.

CONCLUSION

A NEW PARADIGM

Our journey with urologist Nicola Mondaini has come to an end. The volume in your hands is an ambitious text. It sets out, in fact, to reach two goals. The first is immediate and circumscribed, which we might define as operational; the second, however, is broader in scope, projected into the realm of collective behaviors and life habits and pertaining to society's cultural sphere, the most complex to discuss and to modify.

The first refers to the great deal of medical and health information and recommendations contained in these pages, which should always be kept in mind for one's own health and that of one's children, companion or husband. To facilitate its comprehension and its transposition into daily life, even for non-experts, we've tried to simply the material without trivializing it, using the expedient of presenting it subdivided into the various phases of a man's life. For each phase, we've tried to highlight the key messages we hope you take away from reading this volume. The result is a handbook of rules, a sort of "chronology of considerations" along the entire life of a man, to be kept within reach and consulted whenever necessary.

Medical science has prepared an arsenal of knowledge, responses and solutions that covers every possible malfunction or glitch. The true challenge, however, lies on a terrain that's little frequented. In our society there is a veritable gender gap, but of the opposite sort with respect to the one dominant elsewhere. For once, in fact, those penalized are men. While the media and marketing and communication campaigns promote every type of product, practice and service concerning female intimate hygiene and the prevention and treatment of a woman's urogenital apparatus—to a degree of detail that was once unthinkable—a thick blanket of silence often covers the male counterpart.

Not one TV commercial. Nothing. Radical repression.

The topic of healthy and serene care for the male body, combined with a scrupulous but equally tranquil prevention, is completely absent, both in advertising and—and this is obviously far more serious—in public education and awareness programs. This begs the suspicion that the relationship between men and their sexual organ remains largely unresolved.

Working in the background, it seems, are two inexact convictions that, taken together, fuel incorrect behaviors. A first school of thought argues that, unlike for that of females, the male apparatus is decidedly simple, basic, practically primitive. It's there, it's visible, before our eyes, it really doesn't look complicated at all. It's a part of the body manageable with a few routine operations. If its problems appear in a wholly evident manner, the diagnosis can take place in response to symptoms.

A second interpretation refers to the organ's totemic significance. A symbol and container of virility, with connected functions in the formation of the male identity, in reproduction, in the determination of a leadership role and much more, it can know no weakness or lapses. It's there, it works and that's enough. You can have endless other problems, lose your hair and gain 40 pounds, but *it* cannot be questioned.

At the end of our book, we can say with certainty that in both cases we're dealing quite clearly with trivializations and false myths, which can have dangerous consequences.

In reality, what strongly emerges is that the male sexual and urinary system possesses specificities and characteristics that are crucial to a man's identity, and that cannot be taken for granted. Beyond questions of morphology—more or less essential, it matters little—the underlying biochemistry is human and, therefore, quite sophisticated.

In addition, the entire male apparatus and its most visible component, the penis, play a role of sentinel and sign for a plurality of still-submerged pathologies and can thus serve as precursors for timely and targeted actions. There are thus no medical or scientific reasons that can justify an attitude of neglect that, furthermore, constitutes a unique case in modern practices of hygiene, prophylaxis, and prevention.

It's useful for all of us, therefore, women included, to introduce and establish not just a new medical-health paradigm, but a new cultural paradigm.

It's necessary to rethink information and education curricula, from a very young age, so as to redesign the relationship of boys with respect to this part of their body. Taking care of oneself must be taught as a value, for the penis as for the teeth, throat or stomach. If it's natural to use the toothbrush before going to bed, wear a scarf when it's windy, or cover up after eating, why shouldn't you learn to wash your weewee correctly from a young age?

If there are national campaigns to promote breast exams and mammograms, analogous initiatives for the early diagnosis of diseases in the male urogenital apparatus, in boys, adults and,

certainly, in elderly men, ought to be promoted just as exten-
sively. What's needed, in short, is a change of pace. There's no
lack of examples and good practices, nor of effective solutions.

In the last 30–40 years women have undertaken a path of
awareness, overcoming obstacles and adopting responsible
behaviors, which today have all but become habits. The regular
appointment with one's gynecologist no longer causes unease
or fear, quite the contrary. The benefits are evident and tangible.

Why not start from here, then, from this acquired added
value?

On the wave of accumulated and well-founded experience
in prevention culture, we can be protagonists and testimonials
of a process of cultural revision that we have begun on our
ourselves. In such a delicate realm, in a context that undoubtedly suffers from a lack of effective information, the vehicle of
sentiment could turn out to be successful.

The classic channels (education, information and popularization) will all have to make their contribution to constructing
the new paradigm, nor could it be otherwise. The true turning
point, however, could come precisely from the passage to a
synergetic approach between the genders, in a logic of a responsible assumption of risk among allies. A prospect that requires
that each of us—educators and trainers, world of information
and health workers, associations and institutions—contribute
to building a common sentiment, activating personal and
collective itineraries, relying on a platform of shared interest
that involves the family and the most intimate sphere of human
relations. Only this way will the permeation of an authentic
prevention culture become the final result of an original process
of mobilization, stemming from a logic of solidarity between
the genders.

When it comes right down to it, it's perfectly natural.

Who, indeed, could provide the first impulse for a paradigm of intimate, compassionate but serene care for oneself and for that part of one's body designated, among other things, for procreation?

We women, of course.

Patrizia

THANKS

Thanks to Sara Panzera, who with her intelligence and her punctuality was for us the best support we could have hoped for to reach this goal.

I, Nicola, thanks Professors Michelangelo Rizzo, Valerio Di Cello, Riccardo Bartoletti and Rocco Damiano, fundamental for my education and professional activity along with the entire School of Specialization in Urology at the University of Magna Graecia.

Thanks to my mother Anna, for her severity in spurring me to study, and to my father Paolo for giving me the example of what it means to be a doctor. I'm deeply grateful to my wife Francesca and my sons Michele and Francesco for their constant support.

A thanks goes as well to Ms. Margherita Pierattini, to the advice of Sara Tanguenza and to the suggestions offered by Federico and Giulia, as well as to my friends Franco Legni and Giuseppe Dati, and how could I forget my longtime friendships with Filippo Fucile, Sebastiano Giaquinto, Paolo Lucibello, Matteo Becucci and Vincenzo Orlando.

I, Patrizia, want to thank my mother, who educated me to be curious and inquisitive and gave me free access to every kind of book. She listened to and welcomed my endless questions, giving me the key to find the answers. I'm grateful to my daughters for having trained me to answer the endless questions *they* ask.

I also want to thank Piero Angela, because without his programs in my life I wouldn't have had that pleasure in scientific popularization that we've tried to recreate in this book.

Lastly, both of us together wish to thank Daniele Dani for having had the insight to introduce us to each other and make this adventure possible.

ABOUT THE AUTHORS

Nicola Mondaini is a Professor of Urology at the Magna Græcia University of Medicine in Catanzaro, Italy, and a Professor for the Andrology Masters at the Universities of Florence, Pisa, and Catanzaro. He is also reviewer for international uro-andrology journals and has produced hundreds of scientific articles in national and international journals. He is considered one of the world's leading experts on penile pathologies.

Patrizia Prezioso, a communications professional, attended the University of Rome, "La Sapienza." An expert in social and health care issues, she has created prevention and screening campaigns on behalf of both public institutions and private companies. Currently, she is the director of communications for Federfarma.

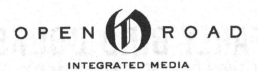

OPEN ROAD
INTEGRATED MEDIA

Find a full list of our authors and
titles at www.openroadmedia.com

FOLLOW US
@OpenRoadMedia

 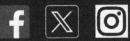

EARLY BIRD BOOKS

FRESH DEALS, DELIVERED DAILY

Love to read?
Love great sales?

Get fantastic deals on
bestselling ebooks delivered
to your inbox every day!

Sign up today at
earlybirdbooks.com/book